Dear Joel
Congratu

This story is for you. Please
read and Share.
Love + Light, Darlene

MW01235554

LEAPING OVER
THE HURDLES OF LIFE

A TIGER'S JOURNEY

This book is dedicated to all those who are living in
despair and suffering due to the many forms of mental
and emotional disease

*"Be like Flo Jo and leap over those hurdles. Leap baby, leap
- and don't look back."*

-S. Sophas

Copyright © 2011 by Darlene Nazaire

All rights reserved. This book, or parts thereof, may not be reproduced in any form without written permission, excepting the case quotation in critical articles or reviews.

ISBN 978-0-9848335-0-4
Library of Congress Control Number: 2011943716

Fluid Publications

*This book is printed on recycled and acid free paper
Printed in the United States of America*

*Book writing and production coach
Dr. Dee Adio-Moses, Healing Center of Christ International.org*

*Book cover design by Jose Santiago
Layout design by Tudor Maier
Final edit by Lemuel LaRoche and Britney Robertson*

The information provided in this book is designed to provide helpful information on the subjects discussed. This book is not meant to be used, nor should it be used, to diagnose or treat any medical condition. For diagnosis or treatment of any medical problem, consult your own physician. The publisher and author are not responsible for any specific health needs that may require medical supervision and are not liable for any damages or negative consequences from any treatment, action, application or preparation, to any person reading or following the information in this book. References are provided for informational purposes only and do not constitute endorsement of any websites or other sources. Readers should be aware that the websites listed in this book may change.

PROLOGUE

How did I get to this point? Here I am, frozen in this state of mind and contemplating the unfathomable. My life wasn't always this rough. As far back as I can remember I was highly ambitious and a pretty happy-go-lucky kid. When confronted with immeasurable obstacles, I stood firm and faced the turbulence. I never bowed to any false gods that stood in my path. Throughout my pre-adolescent years in a unique Islamic commune, to the prestigious Morehouse College, then to St. John's University, and on to work for one of the big four accounting firms on Wall Street, I still maintained my principles and integrity. I've been fortunate to travel the world. I have gained lots of friends, acquaintances, and girlfriends. So why am I here? How did I get this point?

Hold on, my mother is calling me again...
Atlanta! I'd give it another shot.

This story is about me, yet it is for you. I leave you with my life journey as a life lesson. Think about it.

Your unique gifts to the world are yours alone. You are more special than you may ever know.

PART I

CHAPTER 1

GROWING UP

L et's start at the beginning—the very beginning—when I chose my mother and father. They met in 1978, while waiting on the Q3A bus at the corner of Springfield Boulevard and Murdock Avenue in Queens, New York. My father was—as women say—tall, dark, handsome, and a hunk. Though he intentionally ignored her, he was no match for my strong-willed mother. She always got what she put her mind to and he fell hard.

That day I knew they would be the perfect companions to help my soul grow with abounding speed on my life journey. By the time my mother discovered that their relationship was a rebound and that my father still needed time to mature, I was already conceived.

I heard my exit from the womb was forceful. Forceps were used to facilitate a quick and easy departure. The doctor thought my mother was praying as she used focus and concentration to push me out. He'd never seen anyone else do that before and told his intern that he wished all births could be that simple.

Appearances could be so deceiving. My mother bore the pangs of labor the way she bore the pangs of life. You would never know what she was truly feeling or how deeply it hurt. This was a trait I inherently took on.

So, on February 28th, 1980, at 4:44 a.m., I was "forcepted" out of the comfort of a loving womb and into a world of skepticism. I was seven pounds, nine ounces, and nineteen and a half inches long with curly black hair, long legs, and feet meant to grow into. There I was—ready to play with destiny.

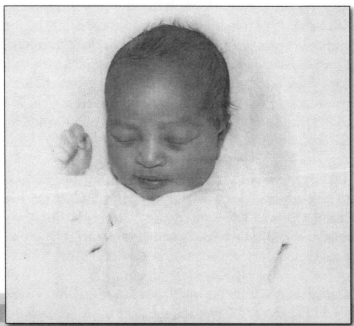

Khaliyq Raa-id Freedom Nazaire, first day of life

I am Khaliyq Raa-id Freedom Nazaire. Khaliyq is an Arabic name meaning "able, competent." These are attributes my parents wanted me to have to aid in my success in this world. Raa-id is also Arabic and means "leader." Freedom is what my father wanted to name me, after him. It's a Five Percent Nation of Islam name, which, translated means "free the dumb." Nazaire is my mother's maiden name. It was meant to protect me from the stereotypes associated with the slave name Jones, my father's surname.

My name was chosen from the Ansaaru Allah Community's Book of Names, an orange paperback that is now a collector's item amongst many. No one knew it at the time, but the Ansaaru Allah Community would become home for nine years—my developing years from ages four to twelve.

Having both grown up without fathers, my parents made an effort to stay together; unfortunately, good intentions don't always lead to good results. Their relationship led to total disaster, bordering on a ghetto-style family feud. No one ever told me the full story, but I discovered very early that oil and water don't mix. I inherited those two extremes, along with the brains of my mother, the handsomeness of my father, and the charm…well, that's all my own.

As you might have guessed, up until our relocation to the community in 1984, I remember little. So I'm relating a blur of dome things that I was told:
I was born at LaGuardia Hospital, where federal workers went to have their children. My first home was in Far Rockaway, New York, which was so close to the beach

that you could smell it. My mother and father split less than six months after I was born, so my mother and I moved in with my maternal grandparents, Audrey and Lenny Hurley. My aunt Anya and her daughter Sha-Asia also lived there.

I never wanted for anything. I was raised on health food, but my aunt Anya snuck me candy when my mother wasn't around. I started school at eighteen months old and I attended a private pre-kindergarten across the street from the house on Springfield Boulevard and 115th Avenue.

At two, I was off to Virginia and St. Paul's College to attend school with my mother, which is probably why I feel so at home in a classroom. By three, I could write the alphabet and my name. I went to a private daycare, paid for by the state of Virginia, and by age four, I spoke using multi-syllable words with a Southern accent. I was smart and well-loved by my mother's student friends. They called me Special K or King Khaliyq and looked out for me when my mother had evening classes.

When mother completed her Bachelor of Science in Business Administration with a major in Accounting, we headed back to New York City. The job market was crap and all she could find in her field was temporary work at Account Temps. She started dating a Muslim guy and, the next thing you know, we were moving into a community, so that I could live a better life. I thought that my life was fine just the way it was.

The Ansaaru Allah Community was supposed to be raising pure souls, infused in Islamic culture, who would be amongst God's chosen 144,000. The Community motto was: "Hold on to the rope of Allah and never separate." The objective was to live of, for and by each other. They advocated noble goals: self-sufficiency, spirituality and black empowerment.

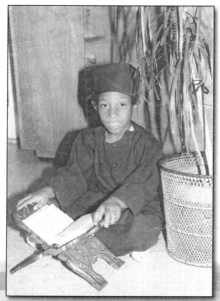

Me at age 5 – Community photo shoot

Community Living

Being an only child has its benefits; you get all that your parents can afford to give and all attention is focused on you. Yet the downside is that you get lonely, and all attention is focused on you. You learn to live with the loneliness and become independent and all that, but it's still hard. So when we moved into the Ansaaru Allah (Aiders of Allah) Community, I was ecstatic. I went from being around adults most of the time to being surrounded by a dozen playmates twenty-four hours a day, seven days a week.

After two weeks, I asked my mother when we were going home. She said that we weren't; this was now home. It wasn't the response I was looking for. All of my belongings were now community property. Boys wore my clothes and played with my toys; nothing was mine anymore.

I know that many wonder about community living. Having lived the experience for nine years, there are some negative rumors that I can dispel. There were also some things that continued to disturb me into adulthood.

 The Ansaaru Allah Community may have been a drama factory for some adults, but it was basically clean living for young children. We prayed five times a day, keeping us spiritually energized, centered and conscious. In the masjid, we recited Qur'an. The music of it was simply beautiful; it took a hard heart not to be moved.

We ate healthily as young children, though you had to eat really fast to get *mazie* (extra) before it ran out. We ate and drank out of silver metal bowls and cups. We ate after the *Sunna* (tradition) of the Prophet Muhammad, with three fingers of the right hand.

After I turned seven and moved to the older boys' *bayt* (house), a daily menu would look something like this: hot cereal for breakfast (most likely Wheatena with peanut butter); peanut butter and jelly or baloney and cheese sandwiches for lunch; and rice and beans or lentils with a canned vegetable for dinner. We traded food like I've heard people serving jail time do to get what we liked. We were growing boys, and we were always hungry.

What I learned in the Community was military discipline. Regardless of my mental or physical state, I could wake up, dress and be out in the morning and be fully functional. There was no lying in bed sick, unless you were so close to death that you had to go to the hospital. You didn't even think about playing sick because the menu of choices did not include lying around. There was no real concept of time. We did our daily activities and went with the flow. I have absolutely no recollection of time-induced stress.

In the community, I quickly learned that life is not all about me. It's a dance of many, woven together in space and time. Success depends on a cooperative effort and patience is definitely a virtue learned. We had a line for the bathroom, for food, to walk to school, and to stand in prayer at the mosque. You name it, there was a line for it.

As young boys, we lived the discipline of being in the service with the spiritual practice of living in a monastery. We experienced the lifestyle of being in a commune and all the gray area that lay in between. All this was done in New York City, nestled into a community within a community on Bushwick Avenue in Brooklyn, New York, in the middle of the ghetto. Needless to say, we stuck out like a green oasis.

One reason that we stuck out was because of the white *jallabiya* (garb) of the brothers standing guard, and another was the *kimaar* (face veil) and flowing *thobes* (long dresses) of the *ummahat* (women) walking up and down the street.

There was also the cleanliness and the lack of crime in the Community. All residents felt safe in this neck of Bushwick. The brothers stood guard 24 hours a day to ensure that there wasn't any criminal activity. If anyone was foolish enough to attempt to mess with us, the brothers would give them a royal beat down. In addition to each brother being required to stand guard, there was also the *Mujahad* (defenders of the faith), our law enforcement and peace keeping force.

We spoke Arabic. English conversation was forbidden amongst the young children. Those of us who entered the community at random ages picked up the language quickly. This left our parents to communicate with us in a broken Arabic/English mix that limited our ability to truly communicate and bond.

By the time I was five years old, I'd forgotten all the English that I'd learned. I, who could speak full sentences using four syllable words before I was four; I, who could tell jokes better than most adults, had forgotten how to speak, read and write English.

From kindergarten through third grade, I attended the community's private school, the Ansaaru ALLAH Primary School. Teachers were brought in from Sudan and other Muslim countries to teach the three R's: reading, 'riting and 'rithmetic in classical Arabic—the same Arabic of the Qur'an, the Holy Scripture. Reading and reciting the Qur'an thus became a natural for us.

Children under seven years of age lived "behind the gate." This was a compound surrounded by a wrought iron fence that consisted of three huge houses. Two housed boys and girls under the age of seven, including infants. Sorted by age group and sex, we resided in a room probably the size of an average living room. The third house, the binaats' (girls) house, was for girls ages seven to seventeen.

When I moved into the community, I lived at 9 Cedar Street with *Olad Saley*, the salaat boys or boys who were of age to begin praying. A caring sister by the name of Naaima Naziymah was our *Umm* or room mother.

Basically, we camped out in a room where we ate and slept. There were no beds; we slept on blankets spread out on the floor. We left the room to play in the yard, go to Arabic school, and pray in the mosque. We played the usual English games kids play, only translated into Arabic, like "*butah, butah, whizah* (duck, duck, goose). Because of our youth, the five required prayers a day were reduced to three, with the *fajr* (morning) and *ishaa'*(night) prayer excluded.

Being from the *dunya* (the world), I was more advanced than the children who had grown up in the community, so they took me out of my age group and put me with the boys who were ages five and six. We were with *Umms* Sauda and Nabiyha. They were cool because they had sons and they treated us like their own, with love and discipline.

At the age of seven, boys and girls no longer lived under the same roof. We moved on to grow into men and women, which officially occurred at the age of thirteen for boys and at menstruation for girls. For the boys, this meant our mothers could no longer visit us in our homes. There was no more *tiffle* (children's) time. Visits with parents took place before school or on Sunday, which was family day. Our mothers brought our clothes for the day each morning and picked up the dirty clothes to be washed, which was done on a scrub board with Octagon soap.

There wasn't a lot of family contact, and it's the isolation that I distinctly remember. *Ummi* (my mother) and I were very close up until the time we moved into the Community. For those children born in the community who knew nothing else, this boarding style arrangement wasn't as much of an issue, but I think it caused separation anxiety for those of us who knew what it was like to have a close loving family. Although I lived the experience every day and came to call the community home, I don't think I ever shook that feeling.

I remember turning seven and dreading moving into the *mu'minum* (faithful young believers or big boys) *bayt* at 680 Bushwick Avenue. All the *olad saley* had to. It was a huge building that had a spook house look. We all had heard horror stories about the poor condition of the house, punishment when everybody was beaten for transgressions, the bullying from the older boys, and sporadic lack of heat and hot water.

Your age group determined which floor of the three-story building you lived on. The brother who oversaw your group was the luck of the draw. Like teachers, some were good and some bad, but very few represented the father figure they were intended to be.

Behind the gate, we had rarely watched TV; when we did, it was a treat. An announcement would come over the intercom system to turn the TV on. There was no profanity, overt sexuality, or depravity. We watched Arabic cartoons and movies about the Prophet Muhammad (such as Khartoum), Conan the Barbarian, and English movies dubbed in Arabic that generally had some subtle spiritual message that reinforced the teachings of Islam and the Imam. We also watched shows like National Geographic; you know, the type shows that were educational and informative. Life in the *mu'minun bayt* was another story. We watched a lot of wrestling and cartoons on Sundays. After the wrestling programs, we'd all wrestle each other to practice the techniques we'd just picked up.

After school, we watched Batman and Ninja Turtles. There was little supervision, and it could get crazy. If you weren't a good fighter, you were bullied. There was a hierarchy based on who knew how to fight, which meant the teenage boys were at the top of the pecking order. I quickly learned that pecking order, and it made me strong fast.

Each boy had to earn his position in the *mu'minun bayt* and I didn't have the luxury of an older brother looking out for me. I came into the *bayt* a quiet and mild mannered guy, but I learned how to fight by practicing; it was like on-the-job training. The fights were part of the initiation to manhood, which were often instigated by the older boys. As a result, I became good with my hands. A temper that had been barely perceptible came out full force. So, people didn't randomly mess with me. My fights were with the older boys, since no one in my age group posed a serious threat. Still, even though inside the *bayt* we may have been sparring partners, outside of the community, we were a united front. They were my *akhi* (my brothers).

When I first became a *mu'minun*, we weren't free to wander up and down the Community streets at random. While the rest of American boys our age were indoors playing Nintendo, we made up games out of what was available. Inside the *bayt*, one of my favorite pastimes was to shoot hoops on our homemade basketball goal set up between a doorframe and a wall.

Outside, there was a large yard where we played stick ball, with a broomstick and tennis ball, and a lot of football. Every once in a while, we would all be happily running up and down the yard playing touch football, and then someone would start cheating. They'd call a down that clearly was not one. I'd stop the game and shout: "I'm not playing no more. Ya'll cheating! I quit." They'd try to convince me to continue playing, but I had low tolerance for unfairness and could not be convinced to play. I carried that stringent sense of right and wrong with me into my adult years. I don't know where it came from, but things were always black or white, right or wrong for me, never shades of gray.

Around 1990, we moved into 709 Bushwick Avenue, a building in much better condition than the one we'd been living in. It had been the home of the Imam's major wives. 709 was located in the center of the Community, which meant we were a little closer to the heartbeat and happenings of community life. The house changed, but it was still a sparring ground.

Community living was more a dictatorship than a democracy. Nobody was overly defiant, but if something wasn't fair, I wasn't one to go along. I was scared of nothing and no one. One brother thought he was a drill sergeant with fresh troops to play with. He had us doing pushups for any minor offense. Usually, I would tell the guys, don't sweat it and just push through it. I even started a new slang phrase: *la tu'ariqun*, meaning "don't sweat it."

One day he decided to pick on me and had me doing an excessive number of pushups, and I just wasn't tolerating it. I refused to do any more pushups and he kept punching me in the arm until I finally swung back. Then I ran out of the *mu'minun bayt* and across the street, something nobody did. No one left the house without permission. My adrenaline was pumping and my chest was heaving, but sometimes you just have to stand up against injustice. Because of it, he never messed with me again.

Another memory that sticks out was an incident that happened because I stole some food from the store, simply because I was hungry. The store owner, who knew the brothers by name, came to the house and said one of the boys had stolen something. One of the house brothers, Baahir, asked who had stolen from the store. My brothers didn't hesitate to throw out my name to save their butts, even though many others had done the same in a hungry moment. Then everybody ran from the room, and I was left to take my beating.

Some beatings were because you (or someone) did something bad and deserved it. Others happened because certain brothers just didn't have a clue how to deal with us. I guess physical force is a weak man's way of controlling others. If not for our respect for our elders, there would have been certain mutiny in that dorm.

We played pranks a lot, too, on each other and on the brothers. It was entertainment. One brother, who came from the DC Community, was named Abdul Mumin. He was from Trinidad and thought that he knew everything. Because he was super arrogant, we constantly messed with him. We had one prank where we booby trapped a closet. We'd set a shelf between the closet and the wall, and as soon as someone opened the door and walked through, the shelf would fall on them. We gave that guy the New York initiation; because he didn't respect us, we couldn't respect him. One night after the lights were turned off, we sent twenty pairs of slippers sailing his way.

I don't know where the money went that came into the Community. In the 90's, the brothers who peddled on the street were required to turn in $100 a day. It was certainly not going to us, who were supposed to be the future and the chosen ones. The Ansaaru Allah day school was phased out and the community children began entering the public schools system from elementary through high school. I was one of the last groups of children to attend the day school.

Once we were all in public school, the Ansaar school became an afterschool and Saturday program. I think the intent was to neutralize the impact of attending *kafir* (those who didn't believe in Islam) school. The year I entered public school, they put me back a grade because I didn't speak or read English; instead of going to third grade, I went to second.

Because so many of us were entering public school at the same time, some had to have addresses outside of the community so that nobody would know how many people lived there. Certainly, our living conditions were a health hazard and a violation of one statute or another. *Ummi* used my aunt's address in a neighboring section of Brooklyn, Bedford Stuyvesant. This was allowed through a special request to attend P.S. 274, where other Muslim students were in attendance.

My world opened up from the square blocks of the compound to two blocks down the street at P.S. 274, located on Kosciusko Street and Bushwick Avenue. Five days a week, we marched to school in military formation by size order. We chanted along the way *shamee/shama* (right/left) and a brother walked along side of us with a whip, making sure that everyone was in order.

At school, we had issues with the local kids, mostly Blacks and Latinos, simply because we were different. We didn't eat school lunch (at least we were not supposed to); we sat out the Pledge of Allegiance, and we dressed in Islaamic garb - *jalabiyya* and *bantaloons (wide pants)* for the males and *hijab* (head scarf) and *thobe* (long dress) for the girls. The girls who had begun their menstrual cycle wore the *kimar* (face veil), and were targeted for being so different. They were called ninjas, laughed at and ran from, so, of course, we had to take up for them.

Most of the *mu'minun* would not fight in school. We were specifically directed by the brothers not to fight in school, but there were a few of us who would stand against nonsense. Abdul Awwal, Hasan Hadiya, Hud and I were amongst those few in our age group. I remember an incident where some boys snatched off our sister Bashira's *hijab*. Abdul Awaal stepped up to them and I was right there at his back. I was a little guy, but I had heart and I always took up for the underdog.

Since I could not read English when I entered public school, my first report card had unsatisfactory in almost everything except math and gym – both universal subjects. My teacher, Mrs. Hixon's, comment on my first record card was "Khaliya has to work very hard on his reading and spelling, Khaliya needs a lot of help in these subjects, Khaliya has to study harder." She never got my name right, and that was just the beginning of people jacking up my name. Ummi responded to say that "Khaliyq will do better in reading and spelling," and she meant it.

For weeks after that, I saw Ummi every day before school and after school to do homework. She tutored me until I made a remarkable turnaround. I knew I could do it and she knew it, too. No more failing grades for me. Over time, I began to excel. Teachers began making comments about my potential, such as:
"Khaliyq is a very bright boy with lots of ability. I would like his work to reflect the intelligent young man he is…I hope he keeps up the hard work. It will pay off eventually."

Ms. Danyziger, my fifth grade teacher, pushed me as well, once she saw I wanted to be proficient. She commented that I was very talented and academically doing well. But she was a little worried about me socially because she felt I could not express myself clearly. Ms. Danyziger said, "it would be good for Khaliyq to work on that. He is very smart and interesting and should let others see that more."

By 1992, I scored in the 92nd percentile in math amongst New York City students. Though English reading

www.youngtigerfoundation.org

comprehension wasn't a strong area for me, I'd made it to the 53rd percentile. At fifth grade graduation, even though I didn't test well statewide, I won an award for reading! I also won awards for academic scholarship in general, with certificates in math and attendance. I was happy at graduation because I felt a real sense of accomplishment. I was smiling so hard, I felt like my chest would burst. My *akh* (brother) Abdul Aziz, was on the stage with me and received an award as well. We may have started behind everyone else, but we'd jumped the hurdle of a language barrier and landed in a place of excellence.

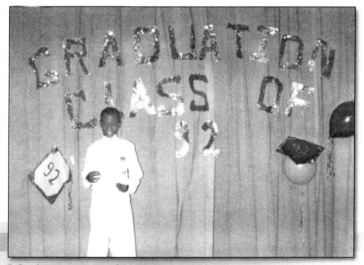

Me, happy at graduation

Going to public school got all of the kids speaking English, and we started speaking it all the time. We even developed our own Arabic/English slang called Englabic. Our Arabic became so diluted that we were forbidden to speak English at home for a while.

The summer of 1992, I had an extraterrestrial sighting. We boys made a rare trip up to Camp Jazzir Abba, the compound upstate in Liberty, New York, where the Imam had lived for the last couple years. It was the first vacation that I'd ever had while in the Community. We camped out in tents, and planned to stay up all night, but I was the only one who actually did. I looked out the tent window and saw what looked like an alien spaceship hovering in the air. I tried to wake up Abdul Awwal, who had been the last one to fall asleep, but he never woke up enough to see it. I swore it was an extraterrestrial mother ship and since Jazzir Abba was known for extraterrestrial sightings, it would not have been a stretch. I sat and watched for a while until I saw the light lifting away. I shouted to the boys, "yo, the light's leaving." I had seen a miracle, but no one even woke up to witness it.

CHAPTER 2

LEAVING THE COMMUNITY

In August of 1993, a few weeks before school started, *Ummi* came to *baytul mu'minun* (the boy's house) to tell me that we were leaving the Community. She said the conditions had deteriorated too badly and that she saw no positive path for my future there. So many thoughts ran through my mind: *What ever happened to adherence to Chapter 3, Verse 103 of the Qur'an that admonished us to hold on to the rope of Allah and never separate? So now we're going to become the kaafirs we talk about and live out in the dunya?* She told me to pack, but I refused. So, when she sent for me the next day, I left the *bayt* with only the clothes on my back and the cool "man" shoes I'd gotten for graduation.

One of the brothers walked me to the *masjid* to meet *Ummi* and her brother, my Uncle Maurice, but I wasn't leaving without a struggle. I did not even know this guy who wanted me to leave with him. I held on to the *masjid* door with both hands, fiercely determined not to let go. I was holding on! My uncle didn't even hesitate; he picked me up and pried my fingers from the door. He carried me to the car and pushed me in as I kicked and shoved to get away. Uncle Maurice was a big, strong guy; a weaker man would not have been successful without help. I'm sure that, to a bystander, it probably looked like a kidnapping and from my point of view, it was. No matter how tough life was in the community, it was still home. My friends, who had been my family for nine years were all there.

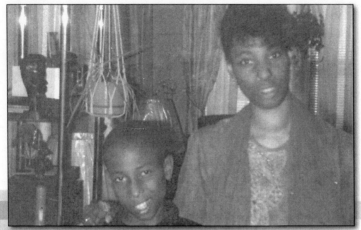

Me and *Ummi* at Grandma Hurley's in Queens, NY

Life in the *Dunya* (World)

It was really tough being out in the *dunya*; life was very different from the Community. It made me feel really blue when I thought about the closeness that I had with all my Muslim brothers and the loneliness of that new life. So many people and everyone is doing their own thing and out for self. *Ummi* asked about how I was feeling and tried to get me to talk about it, but I didn't want to talk.

The adjustment was hard. Though I'd only traveled from Brooklyn to Queens, the journey seemed like it should require a passport. Arabic was my first language; I spoke English, but not like a native. There were many colloquialisms that I didn't understand. I may as well have been coming from another country; the culture shock was just that dramatic. These *kaafirs (non-Muslims)* probably thought I was the slow one, but I'm smarter than the average bear, and just like public school, I was swift at learning the new scene.

The administration saw my birth place noted as Far Rockaway, New York, when I was registered in school. The Ansaaru Allah Community was so far from what people think about when they think of New York City that I may as well have grown up in Sudan. This experience taught me how it feels to be a stranger in a foreign land with the need to quickly assimilate for survival. It did help me, later, to develop compassion for the foreigners whom I dealt with in the work world.

Literally, one day I was living what I knew and the next day I was not. After living for so long around face veils and thobes, it boggled my mind that a woman would basically expose her entire body when she knew that it would only create temptation and lust for men. And why would men desire to be lustful or tempted? It was all very foreign to me. I mean, even the concept of littering your own environment was just insane to me. Luckily, we had begun to wear American street clothes while I was still living in the Community. Muslims were not safe on the streets of New York after the February World Trade Center bombing, so the Imam had determined that we should stop wearing Islamic garb.

In those first few weeks after leaving the community, I stayed in the house a lot. We moved in with my maternal grandmother, Grandma Hurley, just before the start of school in September. An aunt used her connections to get me into a good school where she had been the principal. "Good" is used relatively here. I.S. 59 wasn't a feeder to a high school dropout factory, and maybe half the students

www.youngtigerfoundation.org 25

went on to at least attend college. The majority of the teachers were good and stimulated my mind so that I wanted to go to school. I made new friends and found some of the camaraderie that I had grown accustomed to in the Community because most of the students were from the neighborhood.

Of course making friends in the neighborhood did not come quickly or easily. After all, I really didn't want to be there. I grew up believing that if you left the lap of Allah you were destined for hell. This new world certainly held the promise of misstep at every turn.

Up until the last couple of years in the Community, we prayed every day, at least five times a day; now, I only prayed when I remembered. Since my prayers were not being answered and I saw so much turmoil and conflict in the world, I wasn't sure that the prayers were helping anyway. By the age of thirteen, I had already gone through being fearful of the Creator with the desire to be good to avoid getting punished, to being respectful and in awe of such Omnipotence, to finally being distrustful of organized religion.

More loneliness awaited me when I finally venture into the hood. I walked around just exploring the neighborhood for a while, but once I had made one friend, Little Chris, making more became a domino effect. We kids that lived around the square block centered around an alleyway played together all the time. We were one big kid family. We even rode our bikes around the neighborhood together. It sounds funny looking back, but we just had good, clean fun.

I remember house-hopping to play video games. When one person's parents got tired of us, the crew moved on to the next house. Everyone's parents swore that video games were messing up their televisions. I loved to play video games and was very competitive. I practiced diligently to be sure I could beat any of the crew. I'd even stand in front of my opponent at a critical moment, so that they couldn't see the screen, and drive towards victory. Winning was important to me. Our favorite games were Street Fighter, Mortal Kombat, Street Fighters, Super Mario, Gran Turismo, Tekken, Resident Evil and sports games. Back then, having a gaming system was essential.

We guys were close. When the movie Mortal Kombat came out in 1994, the neighborhood crew went to watch it at the Sunrise Highway theatre in Valley Stream, New York. We made our way through the metal detectors, got our snacks and settled down to enjoy the movie. We took up an entire row. That was one of many really good times.

Around school, there was a lot of bullying, stealing, and selling bus passes. Two schoolmates, Morris and Jamari, and I were going home after school one day when we noticed a few guys standing around watching everybody. Morris and Jamari knew these guys and their reputation for bullying smaller kids. I was still the new kid on the block, but we all knew that they were going to ask for our bus passes. Morris and Jamari tried to get me to cross the street or go another way home. I told them they could cross the street if they wanted to. I wasn't punking out to some bullies. I had learned in the Community not to let anyone intimidate me. If they were going to take my bus pass, they would have to beat me down for it. If I ran, they would just come back another day.

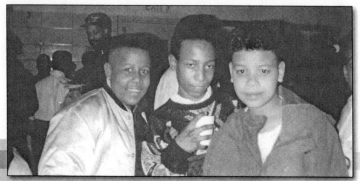

Morris, me and Jamari in the cafeteria at I.S. 59

Those three guys were bigger than us and looked like they'd been left back a few times. They asked me for my bus pass, but I refused to give it to them. They proceeded to jump me. While I fought the good fight and used all my best moves, they still beat me up and took my bus pass. After all, it was three against one. I know I walked into it, but it was important to me for them to know that they could not put fear in me. Once they knew that, the word would spread. Reputation was important.

The next day, *Ummi* came up to the school with me to report the incident to Principal Kerwin. I stood there with a bruised face and aching body and identified them, but nothing came of following the good citizen path. That same day, my uncle picked me up from school and we waited for the boys at the bus stop. He let them know what would happen if they messed with his nephew. Their crew didn't have any mouth then and nobody bothered me after that. I remember feeling good that someone had my back.

That experience taught me that you couldn't have anything for yourself in the world. I really didn't understand how it was one against the other and people would rob and steal from you in broad daylight, not because of hunger or necessity, just simply because they wanted what you had.

Shortly after the bus pass incident, I was riding my brand new, shiny blue Schwinn bicycle and was chased by some kids on bikes of their own who wanted to take mine from me. Man, I rode like a bat out of hell to the house. My mother happened to be on the front steps and asked me what the problem was. I pointed to the corner and told her the two boys were lying in wait for me to take my bike. That crazy woman went over there and warned them to leave me alone, asked them why they needed my bike when they clearly had their own, and told them to leave before she called the cops. People had to really do something to piss you off in that neighborhood for you to call the cops because the New York Police Department has such a bad reputation for racially profiling black youth.

Within a month, someone had stolen my bike from outside the corner store. It was around that time that I started having nightmares about somebody trying to get me in my sleep. If someone tried to wake me up, I'd jump up ready to fight. *Ummi* learned to wake me up cautiously and slowly.

To protect myself, I started working out. My Uncle Chuck gave me an old bench set that I set up in the garage and used diligently twice a day. I found out about creatine and other protein drinks and started reading muscle magazines. At first, Jamari just watched, but when he began to see my resulting physique, he began to work out with me, too. I had to push him. I'd tell him to "keep going, don't stop, don't think."

After several weeks, I was pressing over 200 pounds, but I pushed myself to lift more and increase the number of reps in my sets. Eventually, I could do fifty reps; doing reps of fifty tapped me into a reservoir of unlimited energy, a really powerful place to be. I knew if I could push myself there, I could do the same in all aspects of life. It's all about coming from the mind and not listening to the objections of the body. I learned that early in life.

After I built up my body, everybody started looking up to me. I was a walking commercial. I went from the skinny kid whom others thought was vulnerable, to Mr. Universe whom everybody respected. When I got big, I made sure everybody noticed. That summer I wore wife beaters or walked down NY streets with no shirt, cheesing. Exercise pumps your mind and your body, and I was feeling good and powerful.

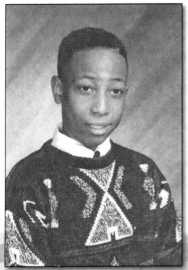

Sixth Grade Class Photo at I.S. 5.9

Even at fourteen, if I was told I couldn't do something, I'd make it happen. For example, once, Jamari and I went to the movies and found out the movie we really wanted to see was rated R. We were too young to buy tickets so I decided that we would get somebody to buy the tickets for us. Jamari didn't think anyone would do it, but I knew they would. I approached this older guy and asked him to buy two tickets in return for a couple of dollars and the guy did it. This incident was a small to show Jamari that the only real obstacles to getting what you want are in your mind. Most of the time if you ask for something, you get it. That's the way life works. The thing is, most people don't even think to ask.

Who Are These People?

I began meeting all these people who were supposed to be my family. It was weird because they knew me, but I didn't know them. The only people I remembered were my aunt Kariyma (Anya) and cousin Rashiyda (Sha-Asia) because they lived in the Community, too, for a short time. It had been really great seeing Rashiyda behind the gate in the children's domain and even better to have a familiar face outside here in the *dunya*.

One day, when *Ummi* and I were at the same bus stop where my mother and father met, I met a woman who said she was my paternal grandmother, Grandma Jones. It was crazy. She was kissing me and hugging me, but I had no memory of this lady. She invited us to come by her house, which was just three blocks from Grandma Hurley's house. From there I was re-introduced to the Jones family. They fascinated me, and I began to come by the house regularly. They weren't aloof like the Nazaire family; they were in your face. I had two female cousins, Catrice and Aieysha, roughly my age, who were almost always there. Though I didn't know my place in the family, they made me feel comfortable enough to find my fit.

It was great to have another family who just accepted me as I was. My grandmother would sit me down, make my favorite meal, and talk to me. She'd make whatever I wanted, even if she had just cooked a full meal. I began eating dinner twice every day, at home and at Grandma Jones's. While I ate, she helped me put things in perspective in a way nobody else could. With the food, she dished out simple common sense. She was a Jehovah's Witness and even though she didn't celebrate holidays, we always had a "non-Thanksgiving" Thanksgiving Day feast. The giving of thanks was for having a family to bring together. She had reared six children – four boys, Uncles Tony, Charles (Chucky), Jamie, my dad, Keith (Freedom) and two girls

– Aunts Diane and Marcia. I think each were as different as night and day. It was rarely dull at the Jones house. After school, I began going to the Jones' every day until my mom got home from work. It was there that I learned to love eating pork, which was *haraam* to Muslims.

My uncle Chuck and I got along the best. He taught me to respect my elders, among other things. Once when I'd rushed out of the house and my grandmother was calling me to come back, I acted as though I didn't hear her. Uncle Chuck came running down the street behind me, grabbed me, picked me up, brought me back to the house and said, "don't you ever disrespect my mother." Not having been used to having those ties, I really hadn't looked at it as disrespect.

Sometimes, on week days when there was no school, *Ummi* took me to work with her. We'd ride the bus and the train to Times Square where she worked for an employment agency that also helped illegal aliens become citizens. I met the owner, Mr. Wilson, and he talked to me about one day running my own business and sitting in the boss's chair. He sat me down in the chair and I thought *wow*. The entrepreneur bug hit me then. I now knew what I wanted to be in life. I wanted to be the man, the cat who sat in the big chair behind the desk running things. I *thought I can do it; shoot, this guy has done it. Here is living proof. Ummi* captured that moment with a Polaroid camera. It was the moment I decided I could be, do, and have anything that I desired.

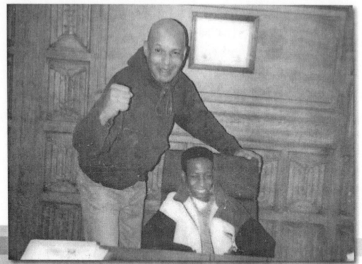

Me cheesing, with Mr. Wilson, Entrepreneur
on a working Saturday

***

During the winter of 1993, *Ummi* and I went to a sister by
the name of Haliyma's house in Harlem to celebrate *Iyd'l
Fitr*. This is the celebration for Muslims after fasting the
entire month of *Ramadan*. By then, we'd both stopped
fasting and making *salaat* (prayer), but we wanted to see
some of the Community family. When I got there and
saw so many of my brothers from Brooklyn, I was so
happy. It was a homecoming . I saw Muwsa, Khalid,
Abdul Aziz and Hud. Who knew that they were just
a borough away, going through the same type of things
that I was going through? After a while, we went outside
and tossed around a football in the snow. It was like time
slipped back a few years.

Too soon, it was time to go and we vowed to keep in touch. Nobody knew or understood us the way we knew each other. We were all outsiders looking in, just trying to find our place in this world. A few of the guys like Abdul Aziz, Khalid, Muwsa, Hud, Abdul Awwal and I did keep in touch over the years. One thing that we found we had in common was that we were all leaders. Our Community upbringing ensured that we wouldn't be content with only coloring inside the lines and being average.

I always had the latest style clothes, the newest video games, comic books and money in my pocket. I'd come a long way from sharing clothes in the Community. I was living the life of an only child again. Looking back on our lives in the Community, I realized we lived in poverty. I know some people would try to spiritualize it, to frame the lifestyle as humble and simple or unworldly, but I call it abject poverty. The Imam had a racket going. I'm still trying to figure out what happened to the hundred dollars the brothers who peddled brought in on a daily basis.

***

Life flowed in a steady stream until graduation from I.S. 59 in 1993. I don't remember a lot about sixth grade, but I remember doing a Spanish play before graduation. The Spanish class was my first formal introduction to a language other than Arabic or English, and it began my love for learning different languages. I missed graduation altogether because my leg was broken after being hit by a car while riding my bicycle. The crazy thing is that I wasn't even supposed to be outside that day because I was on punishment. Talk about being busted.

I remember that my friends were going on to Edison High School in Jamaica, Queens and my mom didn't want me to go there. She decided I would go to Newton to focus on becoming an architect because I did so well in math and loved to draw. *Ummi* wanted me to have a trade as well as a college education. Note, I said my mother decided my choice of high school because I wanted to go to Edison with my new friends. I certainly did not want to start over as the new kid on the block again, but I ended up at Newton High School. Newton is in Elmhurst, Queens, which meant I would be over an hour away from home without a single friend in sight. I despised going to that school. I felt isolated. Again I had to scan the environment for potential enemies and prove myself. I became bored and depressed and started acting out in class. Then I started skipping class and spending my time outside the building – still at school, just not in it. I wish I had known then that one in eight teens suffer from depression. I would have had a better understanding of what I was going through. When we had to write essays, I would always write something shocking, but they really expressed what I was feeling.

Literature Class Short Essay Assignment, October 21, 1995

> *The apple struggles while it's in your mouth and gives off a bad poison (but to you it's apple juice). The apple gives up after he notices that there's no stopping this greedy human. He's now half dead and all he can see is the food you had yesterday – murdered, and he is next. He then*

faints and before he knows it he's in with millions of feces in the Hudson River.

The poem I wrote earlier in the year in April got me thrown out of class and labeled me a potential dropout.

Free styling, buck wyling
on the island of marijuana
kill mad heroes.
Empty clips left zero,
another wants to test his skill.
Ya know I keep it real,
so the body's up the hill.

There was more excitement going on outside the school than inside so I began hanging out there with the cool crew more and more. Pretty quickly, I found out what hanging out with the cool crew got you– suspended.

Since I obviously wasn't doing very well in the maze of the traditional public school system, my mother thought an alternative school might work better for me. The only reason I was allowed to return to Newton and not be expelled from the public school system was because, as the security guard put it to my moms, "We see you more than we see your son." My moms made sure that everybody knew she cared. Clearly, she didn't see that she was part of the problem. If I'd gone to Edison with my friends, I wouldn't have had problems with delinquency. I was highly intelligent and my dilemma had to do with having to adjust once again. My attitude was reflected in my teacher's comments at Newton, which went from "highly motivated and cooperative" (math class) to "a distractive influence in class" (biology). I rarely went to the drafting class. Even though I had potential, I simply did not want to be there.

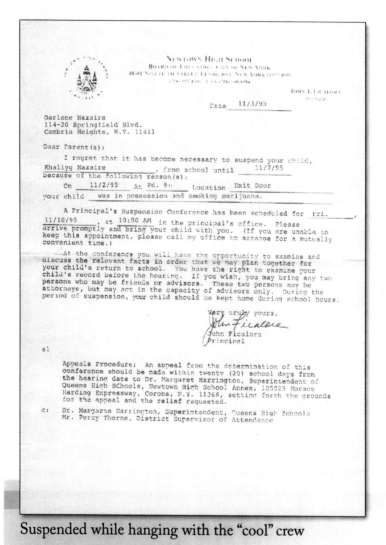

NEWTOWN HIGH SCHOOL
BOARD OF EDUCATION · CITY OF NEW YORK
48-01 NINETIETH STREET · ELMHURST, NEW YORK 11373-9999
(718) 592-4800 · FAX (718) 699-8584

JOHN J. FICALORA
Principal

Date ___11/3/95___

Darlene Nazaire
114-20 Springfield Blvd.
Cambria Heights, N.Y. 11411

Dear Parent(s):

I regret that it has become necessary to suspend your child,
___Khaliyg Nazaire___, from school until ___11/7/95___
because of the following reason(s):

On ___11/2/95___ At Pd. 9 ___ Location ___Exit Door___
your child ___was in possession and smoking marijuana.___

A Principal's Suspension Conference has been scheduled for ___Fri.___,
___11/10/95___, at 10:00 AM in the principal's office. Please
arrive promptly and bring your child with you. (If you are unable to
keep this appointment, please call my office to arrange for a mutually
convenient time.)

At the conference you will have the opportunity to examine and
discuss the relevant facts in order that we may plan together for
your child's return to school. You have the right to examine your
child's record before the hearing. If you wish, you may bring any two
persons who may be friends or advisors. These two persons may be
attorneys, but may act in the capacity of advisors only. During the
period of suspension, your child should be kept home during school hours.

Very truly yours,

John Ficalora
John Ficalora
Principal

sl

Appeals Procedure: An appeal from the determination of this
conference should be made within twenty (20) school days from
the hearing date to Dr. Margaret Harrington, Superintendent of
Queens High Schools, Newtown High School Annex, 105025 Horace
Harding Expressway, Corona, N.Y. 11368, setting forth the grounds
for the appeal and the relief requested.

c: Dr. Margarte Harrington, Superintendent, Queens High Schools
   Mr. Percy Thorne, District Supervisor of Attendance

Suspended while hanging with the "cool" crew

My mother didn't know what to do with me during that crazy time so she sent me to live with my father. She packed a suitcase with my essentials, called a cab and sent me off to the other side of town, South Ozone Park. I was there less than a half an hour before he started with the rules and regulations and telling me that I was spoiled and pampered. He said if I wasn't going to follow the rules, I could go back home. I immediately chose to go back home. He called a cab, and less than two hours after I'd left, I was back on Springfield Boulevard ringing the doorbell. My mother opened the door, looked at me, and didn't even ask any questions. She didn't seem surprised and I wondered why she would send me away in the first place. I never gave my father another real chance after that. He never really stepped up and did anything special enough to make me fully change my mind either. I mean, who doesn't give a kid a chance; and what kind of father, even if the mother says to stay away, doesn't come to see about their child? There was no excuse for such negligence.

In the fall of 1996, I transferred to West Side High School, an alternative school on 34th Street in Manhattan, right in the middle of the garment district and New York City style-chaos. The old New York building was donated by the city and occupied by rats. No matter what its appearance, West Side loved me and I loved West Side. Typical public schools are not for non-typical students. Everybody doesn't learn the same way. I left Newtown High School a juvenile delinquent, but West Side gave me a fresh start. There, I wasn't just a number or a black male statistic headed for jail. West Side students were in a partnership with the faculty for success.

I entered West Side after a year at Newtown with two credits and a last chance in the New York City Public

School system. I left Westside two years later, a model student graduating second in my class, on my way to Morehouse College. My desire to do well was so strong that I also went to night school so that I could graduate with other students my age. I wanted to recover the year I lost when I began public school and didn't speak much English.

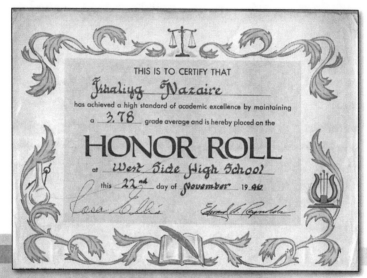

THIS IS TO CERTIFY THAT

Jihaliyg Nazaire

has achieved a high standard of academic excellence by maintaining

a ___3.78___ grade average and is hereby placed on the

HONOR ROLL

at _West Side High School_

this _22nd_ day of _November_ 19 _96_

I stayed on the Honor Roll and became a student leader

While at Westside, I joined the wrestling team and eventually became the team captain. There was no surprise that I did well and won trophies at wrestling events. All those hours of watching Hulk Hogan in the World Wrestling Federation on television and wrestling with my brothers in the Community paid off.

In 1997, my last year at Westside, I also participated in the You Can Go to College Committee (YCGTCC). They made going to college more than just a nice concept; they made it accessible. Though we hated sitting in a classroom on our Saturdays, practicing for the SAT, studying vocabulary flash cards and checking out colleges, I think a lot of the kids would have never made it without the support system offered by the YCGTCC. My mom also played an important role by acting as Secretary to the founder, Dorita Clarke.

Those Saturdays spent studying raised my SAT score on the verbal by 70 points, and another 70 points on the math. It made a difference. Once I went to Georgia and toured the campuses of Clark Atlanta, Georgia State and Morehouse, I no longer had doubts about college. When I saw the students strolling around the grounds, I knew college life was for me. I applied to all three schools and was accepted by all of them.

One of the keys to being accepted to multiple colleges was the package that YCGTCC had us pull together, which included an essay of introduction, certificates and awards and recommendation letters. In the process, I learned how to sell myself. The essay was an opportunity to show that I had the potential and skill set needed to be successful in college. I also had recommendation letters from public figures, teachers, school counselors and past employers. The principal at Westside had great faith in me; he wrote a glowing recommendation letter that I included in my package. I have to admit, it was a very impressive resume for a young man. One version of my autobiography read like this:

Autobiography of Khaliyq R. Nazaire

I am an African-American male, who was born and raised primarily in New York City. I have spent most of my life in the City, and look forward to attending school and living in the South.

I attend West Side High School in Manhattan, New York. This year I will be graduating at the top of my class. Since I started at West Side, I have consistently been a member of the Honor Society. In school, I work part-time as a student aide, am a member of the chess club, and have been on the basketball and baseball teams. I am now a member and junior instructor on the weight lifting team.

Outside of school, I have done volunteer work with local officials, such as Councilman A. Spigner, Congressman G. Meeks, and Assemblyman W. Scarborough on their election campaigns. I was chosen to participate in the Outward Bound School to Work Program over the summer, where I learned journalism skills.

I currently work with a not-for-profit organization called Networking Sistas, Inc. as Teen Director. On the weekends, I work with my uncle's realty company, where I have learned a lot about buying and selling homes. I am also a member of the "You Can Go to College Committee", which is helping me prepare for the college experience.

I am interested in majoring in the field of business finance, and am considering becoming a financial advisor. I have researched various careers in the field, and am very impressed with the many directions I can go in finance. I have applied for a summer internship with Citibank to get some experience in the field.

After I get this scholarship, I plan to show my appreciation by working hard to receive good grades. My ultimate goal is to give back to the community by giving others assistance and instruction. My hobbies are reading, weight lifting, playing chess and basketball, and going to the movies.

Thank you for your consideration of this application.

WEST SIDE HIGH SCHOOL
EDWARD A. REYNOLDS, PRINCIPAL
500 EIGHTH AVENUE
NEW YORK, NY 16018

TEL: (212) 967-7256   FAX: (212) 967-4565

March 3, 1998

To Whom It May Concern:

Khalique Nazaire is a terrific young man. In fact, in my 23 years as principal I have rarely encountered a more focused student. It seems that he achieves whatever he sets his mind on accomplishing.

Last year I had the pleasure of teaching two classes in which Khalique was a student. As he has demonstrated in all of his other classes, he performed on an honors basis. He was pensive, thorough and analytical.

There are many school projects with which Khalique has been involved. He is friendly and personable. He has my highest recommendation.

Very truly yours,

Edward A. Reynolds
Principal

ER:sh

Recommendation Letter From Principal Kerwin

I remember coming home during my first Christmas break from Morehouse and speaking to students participating in the YCGTCC about the attainability of a college education and my experience as a freshman. I also gave them the "you can do it too" pep talk. It was important

www.youngtigerfoundation.org

for me to share that experience. Being at Morehouse was worlds away from Jamaica, Queens. I continued to mentor a few participants who came to Morehouse and the YCGTCC awarded me with a certificate for distinguished achievement.

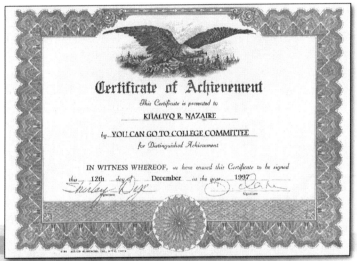

You Can Go to
College Committee Certificate of Achievement

I graduated from high school second in my class only because I discovered girls; actually, one girl in particular, with womanly curves and a love for Khaliyq Nazaire. I had already been named class valedictorian, and then I just lost my mind over this girl. Going to school became less important, since it was the only time that we had to spend alone. That discovery also resulted in my having to attend summer school to get two more credits before I could receive my high school diploma and be officially accepted into college.

That was to be my last summer working with Uncle Chuck. Over the years, he had exposed me to some basic things that a young man needed to know. He taught me enough carpentry to make small repairs without calling someone in. He taught me and my friends how to paint, to compound a wall, and use electric tools – stuff men should know, and stuff that women love for men to know. At the time, I didn't realize the benefit and thought he was a real jerk for trying to make us work so hard doing manual labor. Later, I came to respect him as a wise and caring father figure.

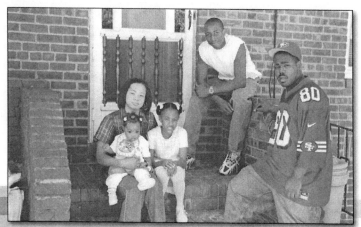

Going Away Party – The younger crew sitting on the stoop. My cousin Asia, her daughter Jada and sister Danielle, with me and Marcel

I almost missed my own going away party hanging out with friends in the hood. I hadn't invited any of them to the party, which I considered my mother's party. It was nice to have family and friends there in honor of me. My cousin Sha-Asia came with her new baby and boyfriend. I was going to miss her because she was the closest person I had to a sibling at the time. Everyone was proud because not too many people in my neighborhood went on to college. Considering my very recent track record, a lot of people were actually surprised that I was going to a prestigious college such as Morehouse.

I wasn't a first generation college student; my moms and a few grandaunts had four year degrees or better. Yet it just seemed that my mom's generation had taken a step back in the education and prosperity department. Some were caught up in the crack era and others seemed content to live off the accomplishments of past generations.

I wanted to take things to the next level of prosperity and abundance. I had read the book, *Creating Affluence, Wealth Consciousness in the Field of All Possibilities*, by Deepak Chopra. It had me thinking about unlimited possibility versus religion. I felt comfortable with Deepak's statement that "Affluence, unboundedness, and abundance are our natural state. We just need to restore the memory of what we already know." Deepak also said "To have true wealth or affluence is to be totally carefree about everything in life, including money. True wealth consciousness is, therefore, consciousness of the source of all material reality. This source of all material reality is pure consciousness. … It is the field of all possibilities." It is this field that I tapped into for my strength.

I had already decided that organized religion was a form of complacent reliance on a higher power. I questioned what most people don't want to ask. How do you know a God outside of you exists? How do you know there is a heaven? What proof do you have? My thinking was that when people believe in religion, they hope that God will help them, instead of taking action themselves. They become followers. They fear their God will punish them; I had no fear of punishment from God, so I feared no one and no thing.

People who have hope and are part of organized religions generally sit around and wait for something to happen. Their God will hear them. A Muslim would say "in sha Allah" (if Allah wills), I will do a thing. "If" was never an option for me. I just did it.

CHAPTER 3

CLARITY, DISCOVERING WHO I AM

When I first arrived at Morehouse in August of 1998 for freshman orientation, I was on edge because it was another unfamiliar place. Intuitively, I could feel that I was in a good place, though. After all, it was a brotherhood to which I could relate. It was kind of like living in the boy's house in the Community. There were rules; there was discipline; food was served on a schedule; there were lines; and the Spelman girls were in the dorm down the street. It was also like the Community in that if you had a beef with one of the guys, you didn't hold on to it. You might argue and even fight, yet, at some point, you gave each other dap and moved on.

I started off majoring in Computer Science like a lot of guys my age. I think Computer Science was big because we thought one day we would be creating really cool video games. When I found out how boring writing lines of code was, I changed my major to Business Administration. The Computer Science classes served as good electives.

I struggled that freshman year. I never had to study hard or long before, so I really didn't know how. School had always been easy up until Morehouse. I was smart and had a great memory. I could figure out any test without a whole lot of effort. So as usual, my competitive nature kicked in; I had to succeed. After failing half of my classes the first semester, I turned it around in the second semester and passed them all. Later, in junior year, I would go on to become an honor student.

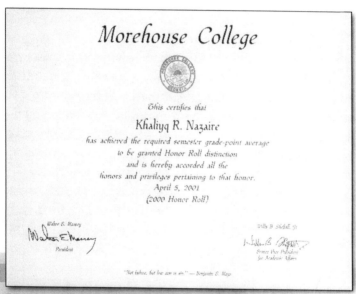

Hard work and determination paid off with Honor Roll distinction

I lived in the dorm that first year and while I didn't make any close friends, there were some cool guys I hung out with. My homeboy Jamari was at Georgia Tech and we hung out here and there around Atlanta. Freshman year, neither of us had a car, so we didn't get around much. During the summer, I inherited my mom's Pathfinder. It must have had about 200,000 miles on it. So, in my sophomore year, when I started making friends with other business majors, we had transportation to get around.

I met one of the first guys I clicked with, Randall Frazier, in the gym. We clicked because he had heart. I was going hard at my workout routine. Randall was doing his thing as well, motivated. As we passed each other moving from machine to machine, we nodded acknowledgement. When I started doing my sit-up routine, he asked me how many crunches I was doing and I said I was doing sets of fifty. Most people do sets of ten to twenty five. I knew that was like saying I only run a nine second hundred meter dash. He said he'd do it, too, and I said, "Little guy, I don't think you can do that." So he jumped on the bench and did a set of fifty. He was like me; he was going to get it done, even if it half killed him. That's how we bonded.

For the next few years we took many of our major classes together, including a marketing class for which we managed to get the answer key for every test. We decided in advance what grades we would get so that we'd both average an A. We used a mini stapler to attach the answer key to the back of the test, and flipped through the pages for the answers. We got so bold that we'd go up to the teacher with the paper in our hand and ask questions. We clowned our way through that class. Just as much as we worked hard in the classes we really cared about, we'd clown in the classes that we just took for the credits. In retrospect, if we'd put in the same effort into studying for that class, we'd still have gotten A's.

As I mentioned, most of the friends I made happened naturally because we started showing up in the same classes, like Gordon and Gunny. We bonded as study partners and hang out buddies. I became a beast when it came to studying. The competitor in me came out and

I had to be among the top scorers in my major classes. Eventually, we made plans to take the same classes so that we could support each other in getting the best grades.

Of course, college wasn't all about school work. Meeting girls who were intelligent, pretty and had a career plan was relatively rare for me. When I got to Morehouse, I was still shy around girls; I had never had a serious, long- term relationship. So I went to my boy Randall for advice. He always had beautiful women around. He told me I was like a blunt force object and that my approach was aggressive. "I'm Khaliyq, I wanna holler at you; give me your number so that we can talk." Funny when he put it like that, but it was true that I let them know I was interested without any game. If they rejected me, I moved on to the next one. Randall told me you have to warm them up and get them comfortable before going for the digits. He'd advised me to "just be you, and talk regularly." Well, I am a quick study and smarter than the average bear. I took that advice and ran, developing my own style and flavor to become a ladies' man.

Females couldn't resist my perfect 100 megawatt smile. Let's face it, I am fine. Mirrors call to me to look as I pass. Even when I didn't believe it as a kid, after I heard it enough times from girls and grown women, I got it. Handsome people have more fun; I don't know about blondes, but good-looking people definitely have an advantage when going for an opportunity in this society.

As I began doing well in school and making friends, I gained more and more confidence. I met a girl named Renee from Spelman. She was the first girl that I opened my heart up to. She was tall, dark-skinned, smart and pretty. We hung out and had great times. I even brought her home to meet my mother, who was living in Georgia by then; something I never did.

As soon as we walked in the door, she asked my mother, "Wow, what do you do?" I guess that could have been a clue how materially inclined she was. I thought that we were destined to be together. Well, she obviously thought otherwise, because she left me for a basketball player. She wanted to live the glamorous life. I didn't have the ammunition to compete with a ball player. In comparison, I was doing small things and I felt inadequate.

I had never experienced pain before or learned how to guard my heart. Someone should have told me about girls who go to the highest bidder. Money had never played a huge role in my life. It was a means to survive, a ticket to the good life that came with getting an education. But if money was going to be the qualifier between getting the girl I wanted and getting seconds, then I was going to have big money. That set me off on the quest for money, and what had been a loosely crafted ten-year plan became a detailed map towards success.

I can honestly say that I've had issues with women ever since. I was crushed, and decided no one would have the opportunity to break my heart like that again. After my breakup with Renee, if some chick rejected me and I thought it was about money, it took all my inner strength not to snap on her.

I went back to academic life holding 95% percent of my attention. I couldn't be distracted by heartbreak. I learned my lesson about the need to apply myself freshman year. No longer was I the smart outstanding one. Everybody was smart, so I studied hard and long to measure above the cut.

Once, when we were taking a finance test, the teacher accused me and my boy Gordon of cheating. She saw him pass me a paper, so there was definitely incriminating circumstance. The night before, I'd spent hours crashing for this exam, so this A was one that I was earning. It was a difficult class and to get a weak B was major. This test was a personal challenge. I told her I didn't cheat; she didn't believe me. I offered to take the test again right in front of her.

The first round of that test, I had gotten three wrong. The second round, I earned 100%. The teacher was so surprised that I earned her respect for the remainder of my time at Morehouse. The entire class was surprised, because they were struggling, and gave me my props. Whatever I set my mind to, I did. I was on target to graduate on time, despite a rough freshman year.

But life wasn't always good in college. I'd get so stressed out around midterms and finals that I would often get physically ill. It meant a lot to me to perform well. When I didn't, I felt really low, got into a funk, and had trouble dealing with the pressure. I never thought of it as a real issue because I always bounced back. I did read somewhere that, according to a survey by the American College Health Association, nearly half of all college students report feeling so depressed at some point in time that they have trouble functioning, and 15 percent meet the criteria for clinical depression. But that wasn't me, because, as I said, I always bounced back once the stressful period was over. In order to avoid all that and ensure I reach my goals, I'd go hard at studying.

During breaks from school, I'd go back to New York to do internships and work with my Uncle Chuck to make extra money. The first summer I came home, my uncle Jamie said: "Boy, what's this I hear about you working out?" I took off my shirt and showed him my six pack. He said: "Boy, put your shirt back on. You're going to embarrass somebody."

The summer of my sophomore year, I did an internship for Merrill Lynch. That really gave me Wall Street fever. It was my first role in corporate America and my first job on The Street.

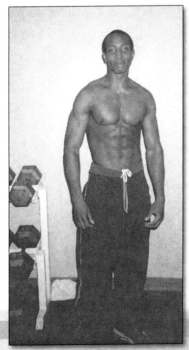

Me in the weight room

The summer of my Junior year, I did an internship for the Bank of New York on Wall Street. For me, that role confirmed that I belonged on The Street. I loved it; they loved me and invited me to come back after graduation in a full-time position. Unfortunately, just before graduation, the job market tanked because of the Enron and WorldCom scandals.

That same summer, I remember my Uncle Chuck bringing me down to the gym to deal with a young guy who was pounding his older crew on the court. I wasn't a sports player, never had any form or fluidity. What I did have is natural athleticism. I played with chess-like vision and drive. He wanted me to hang with this guy who played high school and college ball.

I started shooting this guy down everywhere on the court. Everybody thought the first couple of shots were just flukes. This guy was a high jumper and nobody really thought I had a chance. Once, when he went up for a rebound, I got there before he did and dunked it in with my left hand. The crew roared. My uncle was proud, and I couldn't stop cheesing!

Graduation was just a few months away and I'd been interviewing and studying, and studying and interviewing. I was so exhausted that I moved forward on sheer will. I had a 3.3 grade point average and an average GMAT score of 580. I took 18 credits that semester, did 11 first-round interviews and flew all over the East Coast for second round interviews. I was so burnt out that I would fall asleep in class. The final interview was in Charlotte, NC in banking. Charlotte is one of the banking capitals of America and a good place to be if banking is your career choice, but my heart was really on Wall Street, where the power brokers are and the money rush still flows. Yet Charlotte wasn't a bad place to start. If they had come right with the money, I'd have considered it, especially since 2000 was a really bad time to be looking for a job. That job I was promised after doing my internship on Wall Street at Bank of New York had dried up, so I was hustling to snag the next best offer.

I've found out that people with different names in this society have to be more than able and competent. Having brown skin doesn't facilitate the matter. Nobody spells my name correctly; hell, hardly anybody even says it correctly! Yet I know that I am an awesome individual. I can accomplish all that I can see. Education is the ticket to getting there; it's the equalizer. A black man may have to work harder, yet I was putting all the right tools in my toolkit in preparation. No one would be able to deny me because of my credentials. In fact I had a Ten-year plan and a rigorous schedule for attainment. I exercise and eat anything in moderation, with moderation being the key word. I looked good and I felt good.

Ten-year plan

Year 2	Finish college
Year 3	Get a gig on Wall Street for a firm that will pay for my MBA
Year 4	Become a CFP – make at least $100k
Years 4-5	Rise the corporate ladder
Years 6-7	Hook an international gig
Years 7-8	Go to law school and pass the bar

| Years 9-10 | Work crazy hours for a firm until I had the knowledge to start my own private practice |

My thought was that the young years were for working hard and climbing the ladder. My long-term plan included retiring at age 45, opening a franchise, and then traveling the world at leisure. Having children was in the long- term plan, but if having a wife had to wait until after all that, so be it.

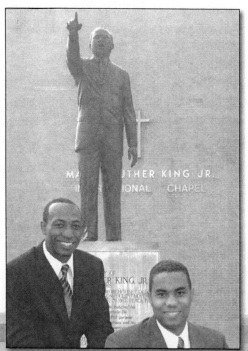

Atlanta Journal Constitution Business Section Cover February 5, 2002, Me and Gordon Johnson

On February 5, 2002, my boy Gordon and I were featured in the Atlanta Journal Constitution under the title "Few Offers: College Seniors Face Particularly Tough Job Market." We were right on the front page of the business section standing in front of the King Chapel with the statue of our fellow alumni, Martin Luther King, Jr., in the background. Even though times seemed hard, we were going to make it. We had to; that's the Morehouse way. Two years before, the unemployment rate among 20-24 year olds was 6.9%; by then it was 9.6% and college graduates were working in Home Depot and Wal-Mart where no college education is required. Gordon, Gunny and I had been really working hard at ensuring our success.

In the fall before graduation, we were in position every morning at 8:30 right in front of the campus recruiter's office so that we could be first in line when the big dogs came to campus. These were American Express, JP Morgan Chase, and Credit Suisse First Boston. Gordon was the fortunate one; he received two Street offers and lined up a job with J.P. Morgan Chase with a starting salary of $70,000 and bonuses that could take in over $100,000. He was on The Street.

I wanted to be an investment banker, too; it paid the most and was at the center of the market. I wasn't going to take an accounting job or something that was mundane just because the market was bad. The money had to be right; $50,000 a year was not enough. Robert Kiosaki said that it does you more harm to start out in life in a lower paying job than to sit out the economic downturn and start at a salary that is commensurate with your skills and expectations for long-term growth. So I planned on going back to school in the fall to get a graduate degree. In the meantime, I'd work for my Uncle Charles if I had to. His business had grown and he was into real estate renovation and flipping houses; I thought he could use a young innovator like me to get things popping.

Graduation from Morehouse was memorable. The keynote speaker reminded us that to whom much is given, much is expected. We had the responsibility to be agents of change in the world. I took that responsibility seriously. Morehouse had been stressful; a lot of work and a lot of good times. I was proud to have jumped that hurdle and graduated with honors.

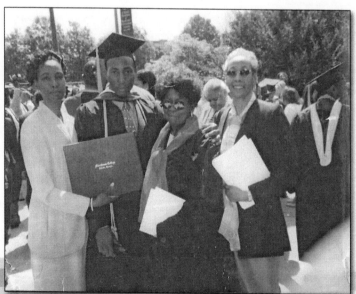

My moms, me, Grandma Jones, and Grandma Hurley

Just before graduation, my dad told me he could either pay for his trip to Atlanta to be present at graduation or give me a graduation gift of a trip to Mexico. He's never been present for any other major event in my life, so I chose the trip to Mexico. He gave me a trip for two, but he couldn't come and nobody else could free up at such short notice. My college friends had new jobs to start and my friends from the hood didn't have the funds. So off I went by myself; alone again, which was nothing new to me.

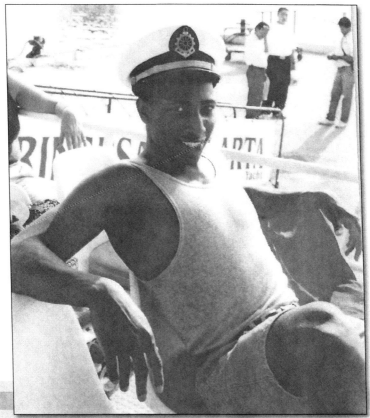

Me in the Captain's hat on a day cruise in Puerto Valero

I put the real world on hold - job, school, whatever; I'd first focus on my trip to Puerto Valero, Mexico. I'd never been outside the fifty states before, so this was going to be a great experience, for which I worked a little on my Spanish. It's almost impossible to live in New York and not learn some Spanglish. It was an easy first language to go after in middle school. Over the years, I also studied French and Portuguese (for my trips to Brazil). My plan was to become fluent in Arabic again, so I purchased Arabic language CD's as well. In the future, I thought I might even study some Chinese; the Chinese are the next population of money makers.

I became more interested in learning other languages when I heard the punch line to the joke "What do you call a person who only speaks one language?" The answer is *American*. Then and there, I decided not to be that ugly American who thinks everybody must cater to him in English. The balance of power in the world was shifting and changing, and if you are not multilingual, you will be left behind.

I applied for and received my passport in July 2002. That started my travel frenzy and, over the next few years, I traveled to four of the seven continents.

***

When I got back to New York from Mexico it was time to make some money. As a Morehouse man, there are certain expectations and the job with Uncle Chuck was not making the cut. It was just supposed to be a place holder and, in truth, it didn't work out as well as I'd planned. From my perspective, he really wasn't open to new ideas; he just wanted to do things the way he'd been doing them.

I came back from Morehouse with confidence and class. The character was imbedded in me as a child and I needed to be productive. I couldn't wait to get back to school. I still got up and dressed impeccably every day as though on a business mission—dressed for the part that I wanted to play in life. Each day I'd go to the dictionary and choose about twenty words to transfer into my vocabulary. I'd write down the meanings and think about the words and their applications. I did a lot to stay fresh and sharp.

Still, keeping a positive mindset of a bright future started to become a challenge. I was feeling really irritable, and sometimes lashed out at people for doing stuff that I hoped I'd never end up doing, like becoming a complacent coach potato. My motto is "Winners Never Quit, and Quitters Never Win". Being a winner is a choice. I chose to be a winner. I used my affirmations to get me through the dark moments, when I felt that I couldn't make it, and even the vaguest thought of quitting entered my head. This poem helped me get through many a day:

> *"If you think you are beaten, you are,*
> *If you think you dare not, you don't.*
> *If you like to win, but you think you can't*
> *It is almost certain you won't.*
>
> *If you think you'll lose, you're lost,*
> *For out in the world we find.*
> *Success begins with a fellow's will*
> *It's all a state of mind.*

If you think you are dashed, you are.
You've got to think high to rise.
You've got to be sure about yourself before you ever win a prize.
You can ever win a prize
Life's battles don't always go
to the stronger or faster man,
But soon or late, the man who wins
Is the man who thinks he can."

Since the work at CJ Reality was sometimes slow and the job market was still crap, I went to work for Account Temps. That was easy work and easy money because they rarely gave temps anything difficult to do. The work was often tedious, like balancing account journals – the stuff no full-time staff member wanted to do.

I also made sure that, no matter what happened, I would have money in my pocket while I finished my degree. So, I also took the time to get a bartender's license and a security guard's license. Security was a no-brainer. I could do it at night and actually have time to study.

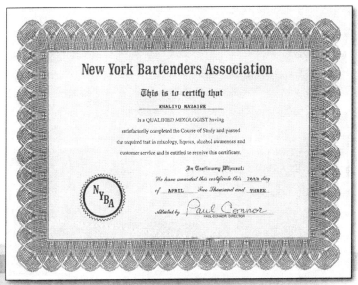

Bartender's Certificate

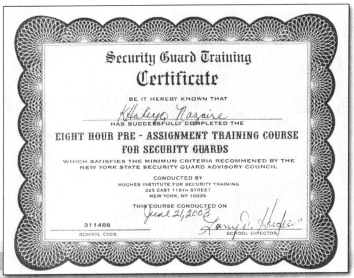

Security Certificate

When I got tired of not having a full-time gig, I went to work at Geico for about six months in 2003. I picked something outside of my field to keep my mind active and to be in corporate America. I was a sales underwriter. I had a knack for selling insurance and became known for recruiting new customers. For me, it was all about thinking from the perspective of the person on the other end of the line. The job entailed counseling individuals about property and casualty insurance, while telling the potential client how great Geico was. I made sure that I was always well informed, prepared and could provide some insight into the needs of the client by cutting through the propaganda. At that time, I was still enthused about the investment world and was looking forward to working on The Street. I loved finance because there is no gray area with numbers; they either add up or they don't.

***

My great-grandmother Dunlap died on June 14, 2004. After having survived breast cancer and a mastectomy, she died slowly from the aftereffects of chemotherapy. Her face would light up whenever she saw me. She would always smile and say "my handsome grandson." Her smile made me smile and feel good. Grandma Dunlap believed in me and supported me with her wallet by helping to fund my senior year at Morehouse when my moms started running out of funds.

A week after Grandma Dunlap died, my grandmother Jones died. She was my rock; her words of wisdom kept me stable. Grandma Jones would sit me down and ask me what I wanted to eat. It didn't matter that she may have already prepared a full course Sunday dinner; if I wanted something else, she made it. She made all her boys feel special. As she cooked, we would talk about life and things in general. After she served up the plate and I sat down to eat, she would get to the heart of how I was feeling and what I was doing. I lived for those talks and the delicious food. The meals would always be exceptional because they were served up with love.

My rock, whom I had taken for granted would always be there, was gone. She had beaten two episodes of cancer, but that time she said she was just too tired to keep fighting. I think she fought for us; she fought to keep the Jones family together. She was the reason we all tolerated each other, and after she was gone, the family fell apart. It was as though we were in the middle of the Soul Food movie, but we weren't getting to the happy ending.

First, my aunts and uncles disputed over who should get what, which caused a halt in real communication. Within a year, my Aunt Diane died from diabetes; her daughter Ayesha moved away to nobody knew where. Aunt Marcia was doing drugs. My father Keith retreated to his own corner. Uncle Chucky did what he could to hold it together, but he was really hurt that his siblings had squabbled over the inheritance. He and his wife Aunt Gatsie tried to pull off a happy Thanksgiving that year, but Thanksgiving would never be the same again.

All I could think was that, back to back, these two really powerful women were gone, and I felt lost. Nobody noticed; everyone seemed to be caught up in their own issues.

Around that time my dad had another son, Kyzelle. I didn't have any feelings much about my half-brother one way or the other. I had been an only child for so long; and I was actually old enough to be his father. What I didn't like was the way my dad doted on him. I had never received that kind of attention, and just witnessing that interaction brought up past hurts. I resented my dad for that, so I never spent time with Kyzelle like a brother would. Nothing against him; he was actually turning out to be a cool kid.

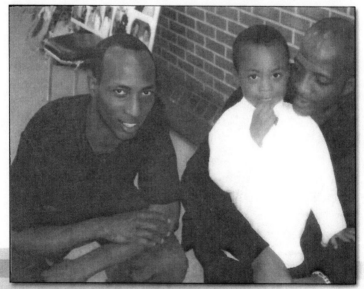

Me, Kyzelle and my dad, Keith

With a heavy heart, I started hanging out and puffing weed more; weed killed the anxiety. When anybody asked me about my plans, I gave them the vision. The ten-year plan was now down to six years and, other than finishing college, I hadn't made much progress. The vision seemed like it was further and further off and I was slipping. I had to get back on my game. So I worked out, read and studied more to keep my mind sharp for MBA School.

I applied to Cornell and Saint John's University's MBA programs so that I could stay in New York. I love this town! Some people think New York is a cold, hard place, but I get a thrill when I think about the money and the power, the diverse cultures, the "anytime you want to do it, we're openness"! My old friends from the hood gave me semi-star status. They were probably more proud of my accomplishment of completing college than I was. Many had never even left New York City and their dreams didn't take them to places of success. Jail and drugs were more the direction. But I must say the friends from I.S 59 that I ran into were faring better than the ones who went to local dropout factories.

While Cornell was my first preference, I was accepted into St. John's MBA program with a fellowship. My mom got me through undergrad, so she said graduate school was on me. Since I wasn't working for a company that would finance my education, I decided to fund my MBA through student loans. It's amazing to me that the banks let you borrow almost an entire year's future salary banking on your success and ability to pay back the loan plus interest. I definitely had faith that it would pay off. So, even though I had a fellowship, I took out student loans to cover the full tuition so that I could make some investments and so that my lifestyle would not suffer.

Just a month before I got the acceptance letter from St. John's, I had been offered a temporary internship by KPMP in their audit practice on Long Island, with a start date of June 7, 2004. I was just about to take the job even though it wasn't on The Street and the salary was only $46,000 a year. Now there would be no need to settle!

At St. John's, I was Dr. Chaman L. Jain's PhD assistant in the Department of Economics and Finance. He was a great guy whom I respected. When I later applied for another MBA program in 2007, he gave me a glowing recommendation:

> *I've known Mr. Nazaire for more than one year as a graduate assistant. He is a great person – highly talented, very cooperative, dependable, sincere and a hard working individual. He never complained about work, and always finished the work on time. In fact, in one case, he corrected on his own the work done by another person, and never complained about it. He always showed up when he said he would. I personally found him extremely helpful to the work I am doing. To me, if opportunity is given to him, he would be a great asset to the organization. I wish all the best.*

At the end of my first semester in the MBA program, I found out that Deloitte was fully funding prospective employees' tuition for candidates majoring in Tax Accounting. Tax accounts get paid, so tax it was. I could still be on The Street, and then could go international if I wanted.

I was given an opportunity to attend the Tri-State Leadership Conference as a Tax participant, all expenses paid by Deloitte. This was an honor and gave me the recognition of an up-and-coming leader with the firm.

Saint John's University

The Trustees of Saint John's University, New York
on the recommendation of the Faculty of
The Peter J. Tobin College of Business
have conferred upon

Khaliyq Nazaire

the degree of

Master of Science

together with all honors, rights and privileges pertaining thereto, in
recognition of the fulfillment of the requirements for this degree.

In Witness Whereof we have hereunto subscribed our names and
affixed the Seal of the University, at New York in the State of New York
this fifteenth day of May, two thousand and five.

After graduating from St. Johns, I headed off for another adventure. This time it was a trip to Europe, partly sponsored by my mom. She was on a three-month assignment in Florence and invited me to stay with her to explore Tuscany. When I checked out the airfare, I saw that it was cheaper to fly to London than Florence. I booked a flight to London instead and planned to travel from London to Florence, then to Rome, and finally Amsterdam. I romanticized backpacking across Europe and bought a huge backpack, which I packed to its fullest – topped off with my laptop. I loved London. There I visited a few traditional tourist sites like Buckingham Palace and watched the changing of the guards. I didn't spend a lot of time there, but I did have a chance to walk around and get a feel for the city. Both nights, I hung out at the hottest pubs and clubs.

From London, I took the high-speed train to Florence. I stayed with my mother for a week at the Residence Palazzo Ricasoli on Via delle Mantellate. The first few days while she worked, I visited the Duomo cathedral, the Uffizi Gallery and saw Michaelangelo's David in the Accademia Gallery. I really enjoyed the rich history of the city. I hung out in the bars that turned into clubs in the evenings. My mother took off some time and we went to Pisa. On the way there, the train was delayed for several hours. Someone had jumped in front of the train and took their life. As a result the train system in each direction was shut down for several hours.

When we finally got to Pisa, there was still a lot of time left before the tourist attractions closed down for the day. We made it in time to climb the Leaning Tower. Climbing to the top took sheer determination because it got pretty scary after a certain point. The winding staircase becomes narrower the higher up you go. Mom sat out the last leg and waited for me to come back down. The museum was closed by the time we came down, so we went to a pizzeria and had authentic Italian margarita pizza before heading back to the train station to catch the last train to Florence.

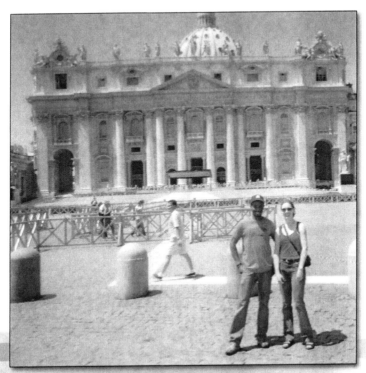

Me and a colleague of my mom
at St. Peter's Square, Vatican, Rome

That Friday, I left for Rome. My mom and a colleague of
hers met me there on Saturday. The room we'd booked
was really small, but the hotel clerk thought my mom's
colleague and I were together so we got an upgrade to
a suite with a courtyard. All that day and the next, we
did the tourist circuit: the Sistine Chapel, the Coliseum,
the Pantheon, and the Trevi Fountain of Good Luck.
Legend has it that if you throw coins into the Trevi
Fountain, you'll one day return to throw more money in.
I didn't throw any money in there. My guess was that
people reached in and took the coins.

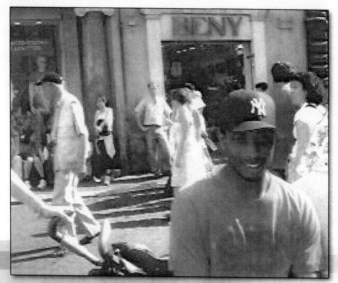

Me, doing the tourist thing, in Rome

I didn't party in Rome because mom and her colleague were tired. I was pretty pissed off about that. My goal was to party in every city that I visited. But after dinner we sat, drank wine and had a good evening. Then on Sunday I was off to Amsterdam and they were back to Florence and work. I stayed in Amsterdam for a week. I hung out in the Red Light District and brought back some seeds with the hope of growing potent weed. The thing that surprised me the most about Amsterdam was that there were so many black people who looked like me.

That trip to Europe was an eye-opening experience. I wasn't seen as a Black American, just as an American, with all the positive and negative connotations that come with it. I liked the European fashions and style of dress and I adopted some of it and combined it with New York swagger. I got a sense of the newness of America. And lastly, I had a greater appreciation for the lifestyle we lead as Americans. We take a lot for granted.

CHAPTER 4

WORK HARD, PLAY HARD

Back in January of 2004, Deloitte offered me a temporary position in the Tax Practice at the Two World Financial Center office. It was a summer job with the promise of a full-time position. After my experience with The Bank of New York, I wasn't going to get too excited about the job offer until it was official. So in November 2004, when they finally did make an offer, I was ecstatic and determined to be successful. I dove into the job of Tax Accountant in the Personal Asset Department and gave it my all. I was one of the first in, and one of the last to leave the office each day. I put in the hours of a senior professional because I wanted to be looked at as senior professional material. Fortunately, there was a gym on the premises with showers, so I could keep up with my workout routine.

Still, I couldn't get over the fact that the work was boring and mundane! It was just as I thought it would be when I was taking accounting courses at the House. What was I thinking? I was thinking that money and a few years of hard work could take me where I wanted to be. But, in the meantime, the routineness was hell. Whoever made up Dilbert is on point because office life at Deloitte was a Dilbert scenario at its very best. I kept Dilbert cartoons up on my cubical wall and changed them out as appropriate.

I worked hard to get to Cubical City and now had to navigate through the maze of office politics. My manager and colleagues had not had half the life experience that I had, not a fifth of the struggle and they thought they knew something about me. They could never walk a mile in my shoes. Their arrogance truly irritated me. Yet they could judge me and evaluate my performance; such is life in corporate America.

Just as I was beginning to feel disillusioned, I was invited to attend the Howard University Leadership Program for first and second year minority associates. All the large and mid-size public accounting firms participated, including Price Waterhouse Cooper and KPMG, with a total of about fifty minority males and females attending. Along with the workshops and presentations, we had the opportunity to interact with others who were having similar career experiences and build a network.

The speakers were mostly minorities who had made partner. They provided insight on how to succeed in the field. They all put a lot of emphasis on becoming a Certified Public Accountant (CPA); as part of the conference material, we were provided free CPA study material that was worth about a grand. This got me even more serious about getting that CPA behind my name.

The conference lasted for four or five days and, in that time, I developed a great network of other associates. Just like me, they didn't see too many people who looked like them in their home offices. It was good to know that I wasn't alone in the struggle. At Deloitte, there were only three black males on the floor: me, Kaliel, and a partner by the name of Jason.

Kaliel and I used to see each other in the office now and then. We'd nod and say what's up, but didn't take it any further than that. We got to know each at the conference though, and became friends. After that, we began working out in the gym and would hang out in the bars after work, particularly Moe's Bar and Lounge in Forte Green. Moe's was a neighborhood institution, our own version of Cheers. Sometimes we'd hang out with two other associates from Price Waterhouse Cooper, Max and Maryland, that we'd met at the conference. But most of the year, we just worked really long hours with little time for hanging out. When Kaliel and I did meet up in the office, it was usually to agonize about the grueling work load. We both agreed that it wasn't all bad though. Some days you loved it and felt that it was rewarding and other days you hated it and felt overwhelmed or underappreciated.

Shortly after I got the job, I moved into a newly renovated basement apartment in Harlem at 552 142nd Street and Broadway with my man and Morehouse alum, Gordon Johnson. It was a nice two bedroom spot with hardwood floors and a tiny concrete backyard that rarely saw use by anything but rodents. It was the first apartment with my name on the lease, though, and I was happy to call it home.

Gordon was doing his thing at Lehman Brothers by then, making long money. He could have afforded to go solo, but he was a frugal guy. That area of Harlem was undergoing gentrification and was the new place to live for Manhattan professionals.

After having had the experience of commuting from Queens to Manhattan, I understood why many professionals were tired of long train and bus rides to work and were moving uptown where the rent was relatively cheap compared to mid and downtown. Our two-bedroom ran us $1,800 a month, but living in the city was worth it.

Gordon was my partner for traveling the world. Our first trip together was to Brazil, which we loved so much that we went back twice over the next few years. The Brazilian atmosphere was both relaxed and lively at the same time, a great vacation place for de-stressing from corporate American life.

On that first trip, we met a lot of cool people, stayed in an apartment overlooking Copacabana beach in southern Rio de Janeiro, and met a lot of "nice" local girls. The city of Rio was alive, with its carefree, youthful party attitude. Any time of the day, you would see people playing volleyball or soccer on the beach and you could just as easily find a party. We stepped into the heart of it and I had a great week there. Brazil quickly became my vacation spot of choice, so I learned some passable Portuguese. People really appreciate it when you attempt to speak their language.

On each trip, we explored different parts of the continent, including the rain forest, the world famous beaches and promenade, the historical ruins and, of course, the many bars full of some of the most beautiful women in the world. I have to admit that in those bars, I shined the most. When we would walk into a spot, the women would always greet me first, forgetting Gordon was even there. They'd smile and say *Obrigado* (hello) Kaaaleeek as they offered to buy me a drink and asked how my day was. Whenever I looked over to see that Gordon was feeling a bit underappreciated, I would flash my brilliant smile and say, "Watch and learn."

Just to do something different, Gordon and I traveled to Croatia in 2004. Our primary destination was a resort in the mountains that bordered on the Adriatic Sea. We landed at the airport in Zagreb and began our cross-country road trip with stops in Bosiljevo, Lokva, Brlog, Senj, Prizna and finally over the Paski Bridge to the island of Pag.

When an American thinks of Croatia, they definitely don't think of partying. Rather, the vision is one of a war torn and fractioned country. But the island of Pag has clubbing on lock and Novalja is billed to have the "best party beaches of Croatia." The Aquarius, Kalypso and Papaya clubs in Novalja were open twenty four hours a day in the summer. Novalja was a wild place, solely for entertainment, where anything goes. Their version of wild approached nothing like what you see in the States.

It was fall when Gordon and I visited and the clubs were only open twenty two hours a day. They shut down for two hours to clean up. We had the beach in the day and the clubs any time we felt like it. I've never been into European women, so from that perspective, the trip didn't quite have the same appeal as my trips to Brazil or Mexico.

Papaya had a bar, restaurant, VIP area, pool, water slide and Jacuzzi. They sponsored all kinds of parties:

after beach parties, cocktail parties, foam parties and all night dancing, featuring different music genres and international DJ's.

Aquarius had different places to eat, drink and dance, aerobics, and a pool. They hosted theme parties, bubble parties, live concerts, and specialized in house music. There's nothing like house music to get you grooving on the dance floor. Club Kalypso was more of a beach sports bar, offering sand volley ball, darts, and badminton. It was a place where you could get fast food and drinks and connect to the Internet. Of course, all that partying got a little old and I probably made more calls to my friends and family on that trip than any other I had been on.

We stayed in a mansion off the coast of the Adriatic Seat. The seaside was so beautiful that I brought two original landscape oil paintings back to the States. Each morning, when Gordon and I hung out on the beach, recuperating from the night before, we saw the locals swimming across the waters to an island and back as a workout. We were both amazed at the stamina it must have taken to make that swim and looked at each other in disbelief. Gordon turned to me and asked if we were going to let these guys outdo us. My response was, "hell no," and we both proceeded to jump into the lake.

Despite our optimism, after swimming about a third of the way, we decided that it was too far. We turned back and went to get something to eat. You know how we Morehouse men do it; we're far more about proving ourselves if money is involved.

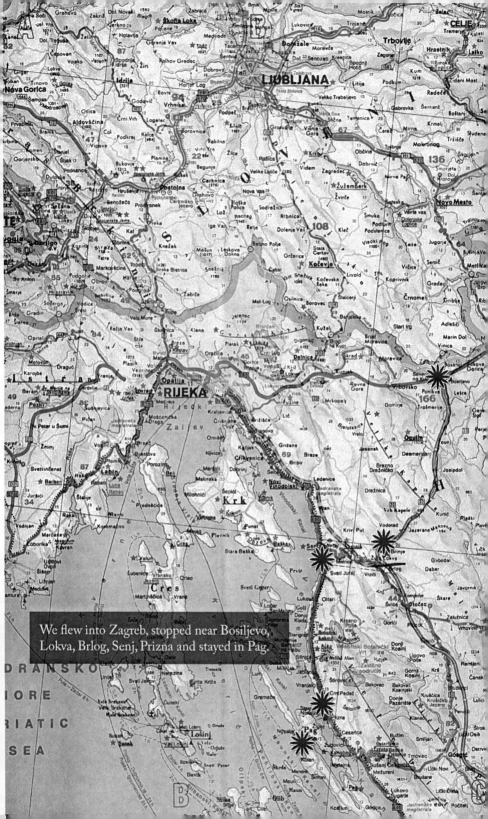

We flew into Zagreb, stopped near Bosiljevo, Lokva, Brlog, Senj, Prizna and stayed in Pag.

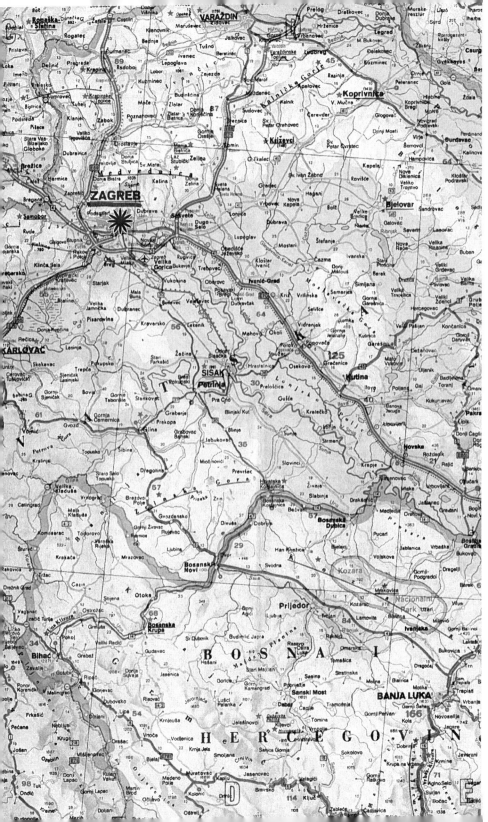

The next day, one of the European girls who was also staying in the mansion told us we were out of shape, lazy Americans. Gordon laughed it off, but I didn't like the fact that she looked down on us. My competitive nature kicked in. Lazy was definitely not a word that applied to me; I decided to prove her wrong. If she could do it, I certainly could. I went to our room and put on my maroon and white swim shorts. I came back out, jumped in the water and proceeded to swim across the channel. Gordon thought I was going to drown, but in quintessential form, I made it across.

I became extremely fatigued halfway through the swim. I started to wonder if I was crazy for taking the challenge. I'd remembered learning to swim at summer camp and practicing at a local high school and the YMCA on Parsons Boulevard in Queens to become the best. I loved the water, but this swim was different. It was like an *Old Man and the Sea* battle for me. I had to rest and float several times to conserve my energy. There was no record time, but at least they couldn't call me a lazy American.

The trip ended in drama. The rental car broke down and I ended up staying an extra few days in Croatia because I missed the flight. Gordon didn't miss the flight though; he had to get back to Lehman Brothers and the grind. I was left to deal with the rental car agency and an expensive rebooking to get home.

Once back in the States I, too, went back to the grind, working long hours and focusing on the climb up the corporate ladder. Gordon and I continued to work hard and play hard, hanging out in the clubs on the weekends and going hard at living the New York life.

When the lease was about to be up at the end of the year, Gordon decided he wanted to be more in the mix and live in Midtown Manhattan, somewhere with a doorman and all. I was really disappointed because I wasn't moving up the ladder like that and couldn't afford to relocate with him. I also couldn't afford to stay at the Harlem apartment by myself. He made the decision so close to the end of the lease that neither one of us had time to find a new place.

We ended up putting everything in storage in an expensive midtown Manhattan location (convenient for Gordon). I had both sides of my family in New York and I would never have to be homeless, but I didn't want to stay with them. I was grown and had gotten used to being out on my own. I talked my situation over with a Latina lady friend who had a place in Brooklyn, just off the Belt Parkway, and decided to move in with her and her son. Having a car was no issue there and her apartment was far enough away from everything that I needed it. We split the rent, an arrangement beneficial for both of us, until my lack of commitment to a relationship became unacceptable to her.

That was the first time I had ever lived with a woman. The issue for me was that she had a young son. He was a great kid, but I'd vowed to never get too attached to a woman with a child. It wasn't in the plan, so I never envisioned that relationship working out over the long haul. I wasn't planning to have any children myself until I was established in my field and had met my early career goals. Since I had nowhere to go, she agreed to let me stay until I found a place of my own.

Finally, I found a second floor apartment on Monroe Street in Bedford Stuyvesant, which was just a bicycle ride over the Brooklyn Bridge to work.

Work wise, things were going pretty smoothly. I continued giving Personal Assets my all while looking forward to the day that my money was as long as my clients. By then, I was into year two on the job and had paid my dues to move up. The next best and logical career move for me was to transfer to the Audit Department; that would allow me to get the work experience I needed towards my CPA faster. My performance review was coming up, and I really looked forward to discussing moving to the next level of my career with my manager.

All of my co-workers agreed that I was doing a really great job, so I was really blindsided when my manager said that my performance was lacking and that a transfer to audit was not feasible. This didn't make any sense to me because I had outperformed my peers. I came in early, left late, and stayed focused on getting the job done. I thought up creative shortcuts to get a task done efficiently and looked around corners. I'd played by their rules, and now they wanted to change the game? No, I wasn't kissing asses and grinning. My work spoke for itself. My philosophy has always been "when faced with a false god, don't bow." I stood by my integrity rather than playing office politics. I wouldn't pretend that an incompetent person was competent and worthy of my respect.

My manager threatened me with termination if I didn't conform to the societal agreement to play office politics and stay in my place. I was rated a low performer and had until the next review to turn that around or get canned.

When he told me that, I had to literally turn around to see if anyone else was in the room because there is no way that I ever underperformed. I was enraged and I also felt cheated.

***

They'd given me a second chance to get it right, but no matter how much time they gave me, I would not bow. I supposed Deloitte had problems because I'd actually used my sick time and benefits. I'd been out on medical leave twice, once for foot surgery to correct painful bunions and then for nose surgery. Doctor's visits for braces took up some time, too. Still, wasn't this all part of the life/work balance? It's important to me for my physical appearance to be without flaw. Medical coverage was one of the perks of employment, so why should I be made a criminal for using it?

What it came down to was that I didn't have the right sponsors in my corner. I was disappointed. If they wanted to rate me poorly, then I'd just stop giving it my all. I stressed myself out working all kinds of hours to the point that my hair started receding even faster than it had been. I started taking Propecia because I was too young to be bald. Later, I found out Propecia has depressive side effects and causes anxiety. Propecia just made my situation worse.

I purchased some glasses in August of 2006 because I was told by another brother in Corporate that they would make me appear less intimidating. I never would have thought that showing that you have weaknesses could relax superiors who may feel threatened. So, even though I always have had 20/20 vision, I began wearing glasses.

I was six foot two, a picture of perfect health and had a strong presence. The eyeglasses weren't totally cosmetic though; I was beginning to have problems with night vision when driving. I wore the glasses pretty much all the time and noticed that white people really began to be friendlier towards me. I wished I had heard of this earlier. It made me think of my ancestors and all they had to do to survive. Wearing glasses was a small thing in comparison.

I also had nose surgery that year. Back in college, I'd had a deviated septum corrected. I had gotten it playing basketball; a guy came down from a jump shot and his elbow connected with my nose. After that, I had difficulty breathing properly. I asked my mom to take me to have nose surgery. As a college student, I was still under her medical plan.

Then, about a year after the surgery, a guy at Morehouse who thought he was a pro boxer was challenging people to box with him. I knew I could beat him and I was on him until he hit me dead on in the nose and caused the deviated septum to reoccur. I heard my nose crack. I put my one hand on my nose to stop the bleeding, waved him off with the other and walked away hoping my nose wasn't broken again. But it was, and though it didn't bother me at first, over time, I guess the scar tissue build-up made it necessary for me to have nose surgery again. I was out on leave for just under two weeks.

Even with all of my attempts to make people comfortable, it became hard to pretend that everything was okay in the office. I'd begun having minor altercations with other employees. At home, I spent a lot of time in my apartment alone, trying to sort all of it out. Where did the plan go wrong? I didn't even want to be around family and friends because everybody was expecting me to be successful. I hadn't even lived up to my own expectations. I'd begun to question if all this effort was really worth it. I was killing myself at Deloitte to be a top performer and my work was totally unappreciated.

Working all day and studying at night for the CPA exam was pretty grueling. In November of 2006, I sat for and passed the Regulation section of the exam with a score of 82. In February 2007, I sat for the Business Environment and Concepts (BEC) section and failed. That failure was an ego buster, but I was determined to pass it the next round. It would be another six months before I even had the time to sit for another section.

When I did take it again in May of that year, I failed again, scoring only one point higher and just four points off from passing. Now I was really stressed. I needed to pass the remaining sections by May 2008, or I'd have to start over. I'd invested too much time and money in CPA certification and continued failure was not an option.

CHAPTER 5

MAINTAINING BALANCE
GETTING OFF THE TIGHT ROPE

As I mentioned, around mid-2007, I took some time off to have foot surgery. I had a bunion on my right foot that really pained me, probably stemming from my teenage days of denying that I had big feet and still trying to wear a size ten. By this time, I was living in the re-gentrified section of Bedford Stuyvesant on Monroe Avenue. I was close enough to downtown Manhattan and the Financial Trade Center that I could ride my handmade Cannondale bicycle over the Brooklyn Bridge to work.

On my block, it was nothing to see a Caucasian corporate-type person jogging and a crack head pushing a shopping cart full of bottles and cans down the street in the same glance. This period turned out to be the first time that I had the opportunity to see New York City during the day. I hit the Big Apple hard, both solo and with friends. My man Randall, from Morehouse, came to visit me after my foot began to heal and we turned the town out. My friends and I went to The Museum of Modern Art, toured the financial district including Ground Zero, Brooklyn Academy of Music, the Bronx Zoo and other tourist sites during the day and clubbed at night. The time off helped me get my stride back. I had no stress on me; life was good again.

The only downside of the surgery was that I could no longer fit into my size eleven shoes; my feet had spread and gained a size. I sadly said good bye to an awesome shoe collection made up of a shoe for every occasion and color outfit. I donated it all to the Salvation Army. Somebody got lucky.

During my sick leave, I studied for and passed the Financial Accounting and Reporting section of the CPA. Without the pressure of work, I could beat the feelings of anxiety. I just needed to take some time off to exit the wild rollercoaster ride and get back to myself. I was leaping hurdles again.

At the beginning of the year, I'd bought a fully loaded dark grey, 2007 VW Passat with a custom stereo system. Though it was my third car, it was the first that I bought on my own. I was proud of it, unlike the hand-me-down Pathfinder with 180,000 miles or the practical Hyundai Elantra that my mom had gotten me in her name. I'd totaled the Pathfinder late one night on a trip from Morehouse to the house in McDonough. My mom took the insurance money and made a down payment on a brand new 2002 Elantra; she liked the bumper to bumper ten year warranty. I was excited about it at first, but when you're in an environment like Morehouse where students drive Mercedes and BMW's, the Elantra starts to look pretty undesirable by comparison. I began to resent the car and treated it pretty shabbily. I was always getting into fender benders and parking it anywhere.

By the time I'd moved to Harlem, I was ready to get rid of it because it seemed to be a parking ticket magnet. I tried donating it for a tax credit, but it caused a rift between me and my mom because I had accumulated almost a grand in unpaid tickets, fees and fines. After September 11th, New York City was trying to collect revenue and a single parking ticket could be $100. All of the tickets went back to her in Georgia because the car was in her name. My plan was to pay her for the tickets once I got my tax return, but she wasn't hearing it. She wanted me to pay then, in case they stopped her in Georgia and had issues because of my tickets. I thought, what difference did it make if we waited a few months? We didn't talk for a while over that. It was supposed to be my car because I had paid off the note. Finally, she broke the ice and started talking to me again like nothing had ever happened. A few months later, we sold the car to a Morehouse student and young friend for the cost of the tickets and miscellaneous repairs.

I digressed there; the memory of that whole incident still pisses me off. This new ride had all the latest technology, including a button to press at the stop light so that you didn't have to hold your foot on the gas. That baby and I got around! No more limitations on getting from Brooklyn to Queens to see family and friends. Unlike Manhattan, parking spaces weren't scarce, and you didn't have to jump up in the morning to move your car to the other side of the street to avoid getting a ticket.

I also found out that women love to be with a guy with a nice ride. Not that that mattered much to me. Women never impressed me because they were gorgeous or simply female. I looked for character and a good head. Otherwise, it was just a good time.

Throughout my dating years, I'd take my girlfriends by Uncle Chuck's and Aunt Gatsie's house in Queens Village, New York. Uncle Chuck would ask them questions that highlighted what they were about. We'd go out to a Korean restaurant in Flushing's Chinatown and find out more about the girl. It was important to see if she was open to eating unfamiliar foods like sushi and whether or not she'd be willing to experiment with (or knew how to use) chop sticks.

Man, I found out a lot by just listening. Later, Uncle Chuck and I would discuss her good and bad traits. I also learned not to be so quick to judge. One time, I told him that I thought a girl was a little strange because she wore shoes without socks in the middle of winter. His point of view was that she was from the Caribbean and not wearing socks might be normal for her. I hadn't even thought about that perspective.

Up until that time, I'd never spent a lot of money on anything except vacations. I was saving my money for a house or other investment. But in 2007, I decided that I had worked hard; I might as well buy only the best. I went through a phase where I kept losing my phone; misplacing my keys, and generally just being really distracted. Each time I lost a phone, I went and bought the latest and greatest one. That July, three phones later, I purchased a $500 Blackberry World phone. At the time, only businessmen rocked Blackberry Worlds.

***

At times, I liked to live life on the edge. Driving fast and running red lights was one of my favorites. One night I ran through a series of red lights while I was hanging out with my man Abdul Awwal in Elmont, New York. We were on our way to Manhattan from Queens. The next thing I knew, the police were on our tail, flashing their Christmas package and asking me to pull over. When the Caucasian officer walked up, pointing his flashlight in the window, I knew he was just going to see two black males. The offense would have been driving while black (DWB) even if we hadn't done anything. So I had to think fast. I said, "Wow that was ya'll behind me. Officer, thank God it's you. Somebody was following me. They fired a gun and then started chasing us. I just kept driving to get away as fast as possible. I couldn't tell who it was. I just kept driving because I was so scared." The officer asked if I knew of anyone who would be after me. I told him I had no idea of anyone with a reason to do that. He gave me his card and asked me to call him if there was any more trouble, then he let us go. We laughed really hard later about that one. But any experience with NYPD has to be taken seriously; otherwise a minority male, no matter what his background, might be going off to jail rather than going home.

That night was one of many when our destination was the Manhattan club scene. We clubbed heavily because my man, Abdul Awwal, was then a promoter. Nobody ever had to tell me to dress appropriately. Dress to impress was what I did. We never spent much time in any one place; rather we'd do the circuit from Club B'Lo, Avalon, Exit to Club Shelter. When we were in clubs, I hollered at whatever woman I found appealing. If they turned me down, so be it; on to the next one.

***

I remember there being a lot of talk that year about 9/11, the terrorist attack on the United States. In NYC, the buzz was about the planes crashed into the World Trade Center. Strangely, I have to say that it didn't impact me a whole lot. While I might be a little obsessive about things in my control, I never dwelt on things out of my control. People asked if I believed that it was a plot carried out by Bin Laden or a conspiracy from within to justify going to war with Iraq. I have no idea what really transpired; I just know that the horrific event was beyond my control. I still found it hard to believe that people could commit such atrocities against each other, and to do it in the name of a religion was even crazier. I was glad I was no longer a Muslim because Muslims were really catching hell behind 9/11.

***

I love the Jigga man, aka, Jay-Z. I feel him when he says: "*I drove by the fork in the road and went straight.*" When you choose to be the master of your own life, you leave the road traveled by the masses. It's not easy, but it's your choice and your path. You get satisfaction in that. There's a particular line from another song by Jay-Z that resonated with me also because of my atheist, or what would be accepted as a Buddhist approach to life if I'd lived in the East.

"*Where I'm from,*
I'm from the place where the church is the flakiest,
niggas been praying to god so long that they Atheist"

Where I'm from, in the Ansaaru Allah Community, we prayed so much for so many years that if prayer was all it took, we'd have been covered for life. Religions have you praying to something or someone that has the attributes of man, rather than the Omnipotent and all-encompassing Creator. Now, that is what should be downright atheist.

***

It was Thanksgiving again and I didn't want to be around anybody. How could I tell my family that my life plan was not working out, that I was faking happy and just plain stressed out, that this life was dragging my creative soul under? In that situation, how could anyone chomp on turkey, laugh and smile and be around people? I'd just sleep until I had to show up back at work. Thanksgivings had never been right since my Grandmother Jones passed anyway. I missed her deeply, so the day already had a bleak pall.

That afternoon, someone kept ringing my doorbell and interrupting my plan of isolation. Then the phone started ringing persistently. Finally, I took a sneak peak out the window. It was my uncle Reese, Aunt Anya, and Mom. I let them ring that bell and call on the phone as much as they liked. I wasn't being social that day.

Of course, isolation was not in the ten-year plan. I'd slipped on my goal dates, so I needed to double up; there had to be another way to get there. I'd work harder. I was studying for the CPA exam and for the LSAT at the same time. I had to keep my opportunities open and someone with a law degree who was also a certified accountant could get paid! In the meantime, I needed to leave Deloitte before I hurt somebody. They just made me angry. It seemed that my chance of success based on merit was hopeless. I wasn't a round peg to be squeezed into a square hole! Since I would never be, I needed to find another way. My thought process has always been "when faced with a false god, don't bow." Corporate America is a false god, with its own dysfunctional culture. I wasn't bowing.

I called my mom to get her advice; she seemed to be okay with leaping through these corporate hurdles. She told me: "It's just a game and when you take it too personally, you get caught up in it, and that's experience talking. Understand your goals, and as long as the job is moving you in the direction of your goals, stay with it. Don't leave until you have your next step planned. Sometimes you have to zigzag to get to your goal. Since you've got almost a year before the next review and potential firing, you've got plenty of time to plan your next move."

I thought about it and hung up the phone thinking that it sounded good. What she didn't realize that coming into the office every day was making me physically ill and that watching people who are half as competent get the jobs that I applied for was downright demeaning. Life is tough for a black man in corporate America. It's like a fish swimming upstream, fighting hard to go against the flow and if the flow doesn't turn, you just get tired after a while. I was tired and finally left Deloitte in May 2007. They offered me a two-month severance package and I was qualified to receive unemployment benefits. I also opted in on the COBRA, which would kick in in November, to make sure that I had health insurance coverage.

***

I had to recalibrate the plan. I was now into year five. There was a lot to do in half the time and there had to be another way to get there. To start, I moved in with my Grandma Hurley to save some money. Unemployment was only paying $405 a month. I got the idea of living with family from a West Indian chick I dated. Think about this; she made the same money I did, but her cost of living was so low that she had bank. It was only going to be temporary because I'd decided to go to MBA School full-time. I had my eye set on Dartmouth and would be relocating there.

Almost immediately, Grandma Hurley and I went back to our adversarial relationship. She'd say the color was blue and I'd say it was red. We'd get into shouting matches because she didn't want to acknowledge that I was grown. I'd been living on my own for several years, and I wasn't going back into child mode. We argued about the renovations I was doing. The house needed painting, roof repair and various other minor repairs to get it into decent condition. I began doing the work with my money, with the understanding that the expense was in lieu of rent. Somehow, she didn't remember making that agreement. I guess she only let me stay there because she needed the extra money. It seemed that it's always about money with everybody. But I was sure my mother was giving my grandmother money every month, so why did I need to give her money and do renovations too? I didn't get her. I challenged her to do more with her life than watch television and smoke cigarettes. Our relationship was rocky. Then again, I had a rocky relationship with most of the people I really cared about because, like I expected a lot from myself, I expect a lot from them. They often let me down.

This was the revised plan: I'd take a job where the so called "work/life" balance wasn't seesawed on the work side. That way I could have the time to study for the remaining sections of the CPA I'd yet to pass. The Business Environment and Concepts (BEC) section had been elusive and I hadn't taken the Audit section. Then I'd go back to school to get an MBA from one of the top four colleges. A Master of Science just didn't hold the same value as an MBA from one of the top ten schools, and didn't earn you the same cheddar either.

When I interviewed at Grant Thornton in June of 2007, I made it clear that I was looking for a job that would allow me the time to study to pass the CPA. I let the interviewer know that I was not looking for something as intense as my experience at Deloitte. I even asked, "I wonder if there is a place for me here with those caveats?" I aced their interview questions and followed through with a few of my own:

> *How does this firm distinguish itself from the other "Big Four" firms?*
>
> *What would the balance between my personal and professional life be?*
>
> *Can you tell me about this firm's attitude toward flexible work schedules?*
>
> *How would you describe the culture here?*
>
> *Could you discuss your progress within the firm? Is that what I can expect if I came here?*

If there were on thing you wish the firm could improve upon, what would it be?

What is the largest problem facing this tax department now?

What skills are especially important for someone in this position?

I made my priorities clear. I needed flexible time so that I could study for the CPA exam. When and if I decided to stay at Grant Thornton and go hard at this tax thing, then I expected to be promoted and compensated accordingly. At the same time, I would ensure that I was a valued contributor working smartly on the right things. With all of that, they still loved me and offered me a job that same week as a Tax Senior Associate, making $80,000 a year with a $5,000 advance on future earnings.

Before starting the new job, I planned a short get away from New York. At the end of August 2007, I took my young cousins Marcel and Jada to Georgia for a week's stay with my mother, with the full trip for all three of us sponsored by her. I had never been around them or any little kids for more than a few hours. They were very interesting, to say the least. It was their first time flying, so I was happy to have that first experience with them and to bond.

The vacation was very relaxing and a lot of fun. We did things like horseback riding, spent a day at Stone Mountain, and went bike riding. These were things I never got to do as a child living in a commune. I kept thinking that I missed out on a lot in my childhood and this vacation reinforced my belief that my mother had been a bad mother. As I headed back to New York with my cousins, I was conflicted between having enjoyed the trip and resenting not having had a normal childhood.

***

After a few weeks break between happily leaving Deloitte and starting at Grant Thornton, I got into the new job. It looked and felt like a smaller version of Deloitte. So I thought *looks like a duck, quacks like a duck … it's a duck!* Plus, everywhere you go, problems follow you if you have not resolved the underlying issue, and the underlying issue here was that accounting is boring and mundane. It was downright depressing and sent me into a spiral of more mind mantras, like:

> *Am I ever going to get to a place that fits? Do I really have what it takes to make it? Maybe I'm just posturing. You know, what is a guy like me even doing here? Not enough, not enough, not enough eating at me.*

Weeks later, my new manager started requesting that I work more hours. I reminded him of the verbal agreement we had when I was hired on; I was not going to work extra hours so that I could have time to study for the CPA exam. He stated that he needed me; and I stated that I was not going to work myself into stress and heart attack. I'd done enough of that at Deloitte and swore never to work that hard for someone else again. He didn't waver from his position, so I quit the job. I didn't discuss it with anyone; I just gave notice and quit.

A week later, the results came back on the CPA exam. I was three points short of passing the Business Environment and Concepts section. The cloud that loomed over me was so heavy; I felt that I just couldn't get from under it. I started to wonder if this depression was a real issue or just a passing mood. I knew that it was in my family medical history. It's like you act out things passed down in your genes that you have no control over. You don't want to do it, but you simply can't help it. But really, I'm stronger than genetics and I worked hard to create a new path in the world.

I found out that this poem is true:

> *I bargained with life for a penny*
> *And life would pay no more.*
> *However I begged at evening,*
> *When I counted my scanty store.*
>
> *For life is a just employer.*
> *He gives you what you ask.*
> *But once you have set the wages,*
> *Why, you must bear the task.*
>
> *I worked for a menial's hire*
> *Only to learn, dismayed*
> *That any wage I had asked of life,*
> *Life would have willingly paid*

CHAPTER 6

THE BACKLASH OF CHOOSING TO BE AUTHENTIC

I am Khaliyq Nazaire; and I wondered if I would be having these problems in life if my name were Richard Jones. I couldn't change my last name, but I could use my middle initial and I'd be Rich Nazaire. That's what I wanted to be anyway—rich! Rich so that I could help my family to never have to struggle again; rich so that we didn't have to deal with ghetto thugs and people always trying to take from us. At the same time, I couldn't conform to what society thought I should be. I would continue steadily on the path towards my goals. I knew that I'd made my life harder by swimming in a direction opposite of what society would expect of me, opposite of what even some well-meaning friends and family thought I should be going. People looked up to me, yet the only difference between me and them was that I had measurable goals, a plan of action to get there, and a time frame.

The year 2007 held a series of bad experiences for me. That May, I tried to help an old friend from the hood see the faultiness in his logic which kept him stuck in a lifestyle of poverty. I was like, "Think about it; if you got an education, you could get up out of the hood." He thought that I was trying to make him look bad in front of the rest of the crew. He thanked me by hitting me in the head with a rock. I realized from the experience that most people don't think. I had simply asked him to think about how he was living. "Think about it" was one of my favorite expressions. I always invited everyone to think about a situation because looking at different aspects helps you make better choices. Who wouldn't want to make better choices? Well, my lesson learned was never to debate with a fool. I had no idea that some people didn't want to hear about anything that expanded their awareness.

I called 9-1-1 and the ambulance took so long to come, I ending up driving myself to the hospital. I have zero tolerance for stupid people, but I called the police instead of trying to settle this myself. After all, I'm a Morehouse man. We do things the right way; no need for street justice. So I did the "right" thing and the police never even followed up on the incident. I mean I gave them the guy's name and address, description, everything and *nada* (nothing). That's the hood life.

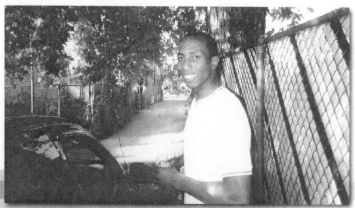

I had a serious knot on the side of my head from that rock.

***

Back in October of 2006, I started day trading with E*TRADE Securities to develop a second source of income. My initial trades were in pharmaceuticals, electronics, and technology. I also had success with Google, Blockbuster and Netflix. It was fast paced and exciting. My peak day was a purchase of $30,000 in securities, which was pretty significant for a 26 year old. Until July 2007, I was on a roll, making a few thousand here and there, definitely not getting rich with it. In July, my trades lost 80% of their value, a loss of about $17,000. That seriously stressed me out. The possibility of failure and throwing my money down the drain in trades was not an option.

I spent the month of August scrambling to make my money back and ending up about $2,000 over where I was the previous June, but that took a lot of time and effort. I stayed holed up in my room trading day and night. In September, I continued the uptrend, but I decided to get out. At the end of the day, I'd purchased $341,000 in securities and sold $344,000. All of that work for only $3,000. I'd leave day trading to those who knew how to do it.

That was another experience I ended up jumping successfully. Just barely; I hit the hurdle on that one, but left it standing. In my mind, I was thinking:

> *"I'm weary of jumping over hurdles. I'm looking back, and this is not the way I planned my life to be. I am competent and able, and it just doesn't feel like enough.*

I'm supposed to be the man, running things, and now I just feel like I'm on an eternal treadmill of self-sabotage. Two steps forward, one step back. If I could get rid of the repetitive thoughts of despair running through my mind, I could shake this feeling of hopelessness. If I can get to tomorrow, I know it will be better. I'll give it a shot another day, right now I'll just go to sleep."

***

I had been saving up money to tide me over while I went back to school for my MBA. After quitting Grant Thornton, I joined the Consortium for Graduate Study in Management to enhance my chances of getting into one of the top schools. I checked them out and was impressed by their charter:

"The Consortium for Graduate Study in Management is the country's preeminent organization for promoting diversity and inclusion in American business. Through an annual competition, The Consortium awards merit-based, full-tuition fellowships to America's best and brightest candidates. In conjunction with our member schools, sponsoring companies, and our elite group of MBA students and alumni, The Consortium has built a 44 year legacy of fostering inclusion and changing the ethnic and cultural face of American business."

My plan was to get one of those scholarships. I had over $40,000 saved - $20,000 in cash savings and another $20,000 in 401(k). My interview skills were outstanding. In fact, at Morehouse I taught several of my peers how to interview and suggested they read the book *What Color is*

Your Parachute. Getting the job was easy. Getting a job that I could get excited about going to every day was the challenge.

I wasn't getting up to go to work in the morning, so sooner or later my grandmother would figure out that I quit. I didn't say anything about it because it was depressing that I wasn't getting things right.

Just after Thanksgiving 2007, I took the Business Environment and Concepts section of the CPA again for the third time. I had a really good feeling and was sure I had finally passed it. I just had to wait for the results.

***

Then my grandmother asked me to leave. She was putting me out. We didn't get along and had been arguing over big and little things. She objected to my girlfriend Kiri spending time at the house, saying that I was disrespecting her. It got so bad that she told me that Kiri could not use the bathroom. I called my mom to talk some reason into her. Really, how could someone not be allowed to use the bathroom?

That December, I seriously began thinking about taking my life.

> *What is the point of being here if life is such a struggle? If those who are supposed to love you will put you out and not give you a chance. What kind of a grandmother does not give her grandson a chance? She had no idea of what I was struggling with.*

Again, I hibernated in the house, refusing social contact. I'd already quit my job, so I had no occupation to head off to each day. I still got up and dressed as though I had business to deal with, but I began sleeping more than usual. I'd often awaken in the early morning hours exhausted from the thoughts that I couldn't even escape in my sleep, and a reoccurring dream that I was fighting someone or something off. Whenever someone knocked on the door, I'd jump up from the dream, ready to defend myself. It seemed things had never gotten right after my grandmother died in 2004.

On December 3, 2007, I wrote a suicide note: *Know when to quit.* I signed it. My mom called just as I was contemplating the act and asked if I was still coming to Georgia to stay until I was accepted into MBA School. She had bought tickets for us to see the Miami Heat play the Hawks at Philips Arena. She wanted to know if I was going to make it in time for the game, or if she should invite someone else. Right then and there, I decided to give life another chance. Maybe she could help me; at any rate, I wanted to see her.

I moved everything I wanted to keep to Atlanta. Because I left in such a hurry, I simply threw away everything that wasn't needed. I attempted to give some things to my grandmother, but she said she didn't want them. I was sure she could use some of the things, so I stashed small items in places she wouldn't notice immediately. The bulk of the stuff, I just put out on garbage day. Somebody got lucky. Hopefully, it was somebody who needed the stuff.

I told my girlfriend Kiri that I was moving to Georgia and would probably never see her again. I shut her out and cut all ties with her. It wasn't that she had ever did anything wrong. She was there for me when I had foot surgery and when I came back from Croatia disheartened, but I never told her about the shadow thoughts.

On December 4th, I'd packed up my car and gotten on the road. I'd bought a bike rack for the roof of the car and strapped on my Cannondale. The drive to Georgia was an irritating thousand mile journey. The wind whistling through that bike rack made an unbearable noise the whole trip. I stopped a few times on the road, making it a two-day trip, so that it wouldn't be so stressful. I arrived in Georgia the day before the game on December 5th. My belongings had arrived the day before and I quickly settled in to my mom's house out in the boonies of McDonough.

I had forgotten how quiet and peaceful it was. It was really strange when I first arrive from New York City and it began to get to me. I didn't run up and down the highway between Atlanta and McDonough because the days were short and I didn't like driving at night. To keep myself occupied when I wasn't studying or reading, I bought a PlayStation 3, several games and a headset that ran me about $800. I began competing internationally.

My plan for the time off in Georgia, before going to MBA School, was to play golf and study for the Certified Financial Accountant (CFA) Level 1 exam, as well as complete the two remaining sections of the CPA exam. I was looking at other options as well, in the event that I didn't get into one of the top four schools in 2009. I was searching for a job with money versus the boring real estate that I had begun doing with my Uncle Chuck.

My end goal was to become an entrepreneur, since few people get truly rich working for someone else. I thought one way to do that would be to find investors who needed someone to market their product. As their marketing consultant, I would set up meetings with distributors – the big chain franchises like Wal-Mart or Toys R Us. I was keeping my options open.

I stayed with my mother for about two weeks before my boy Randall convinced me that it was not cool to be grown and living with your mother. He had a nice crib over on the south side, so I decided to rent a room from him until I went to MBA School. After all, my mother wasn't letting me stay there free; she wanted me to take on a major bill. Everybody wants your money. I gave her a grand to show her that money wasn't an issue.

Life at Randall's wasn't the camaraderie that I'd expected and needed. He worked long hours and stayed with his girlfriend a lot, so I was often alone. It seemed as though bad luck had followed me from New York. First my car was sideswiped, leaving a streak of white paint on the driver's side of my new ride. Then I got the news that I failed the BEC section of the CPA exam again, this time by one point. That really depressed me. I didn't think I could have studied any harder than I did before taking that exam. I moped around for a week after that. When I went to visit my mom, I couldn't shake the depression. I told her that I had failed the exam. She responded by saying, "Well, I know that you're not letting a test get you down like that. Stay focused, you can do anything you want to do." As I opened the refrigerator door looking for something to eat, I just sighed heavily, thinking *if only she knew.*

Randall didn't have a high tech TV for gaming, so I went out and bought a 42" flat screen Samsung so that I could whoop him. Internet gaming is cool, but it's better to beat someone in person. In addition to online gaming, I started online dating, meeting up with the girls in different hot spots around the Atlanta area for entertainment.

Between doing CPA and Law School Admission Test (LSAT) practice exams, gaming and online dating, I was spending a lot of time on the computer. I didn't have much else to do as I waited for the results of my application to MBA School. I wasn't happy and it was hard to stay busy.

By New Year's Eve, I'd begun working my way back to a place of peace. I made peace with my demons and with God. I had New Year's Day dinner with family and friends at my mom's house. There was good food and the conversation flowed nicely. We were a motley crew: me, my mom, Randall and his girlfriend, and my mom's friend Raina and her girlfriend Lavonne. Lavonne was also an accountant so we bonded and talked shop.

Everybody was a couple except me and my mom. I felt a little envious of the relationship Randall had with his girl. They had discussed marriage and seemed to be an ideal Morehouse/Spelman couple. I didn't have anybody in my life like that. I'd had many girlfriends but the ones who I thought would be special, like Renee, didn't pan out. The ones who wanted to be special just didn't meet my criteria for a wife. But I wasn't worried about all that that day; I was relaxed and having a good time. I had some wine for the first time in over a year. I'd sworn off alcohol the previous New Year's Day and hadn't touched it since. But everybody was having a good time and I felt up to partaking.

***

I should have never started drinking again. Now that I'd broken the discipline, I was drinking in the evenings and tipsy before I even got out on the town. Randall was into drinking Jack Daniels and I'd been tapping into his stash. Strong stuff, but I needed strong stuff to help quiet the pain and paranoia I felt.

I had always felt the need to carry protection. In New York, a legal gun was hard to get. In Georgia, it seemed anybody who was of age and had the proper ID could get a gun. One evening, I went into the Georgia Range and Guns store in Forest Park with the intention of buying a handgun. The guy behind the counter did an upsell and offered me a discount on a second gun. The feel of the metal gave me a rush of excitement. I bought a .45 caliber Kimber Custom TLE II pistol and a Spring Micro pistol, each for about a thousand dollars, and some .45 caliber bullets. Finally, I was a gun owner. The next day, I started going to the range for target practice. There was a shooting range right down the road from Randall's crib. I was good at it. In fact, I enjoyed it so much that I tried to get Randall to come with me to share the experience.

I'd been talking to Randall about the shadow self I'd been experiencing. Over the past few years, it seemed like when I got stressed, a dark side of my personality would come out, and I was beginning to have power to control it. In college, I had shared with him how I felt paranoid at times, so he knew that I sometimes struggled. Nobody else knew. I might have thrown it out there to other people by telling them that I was paranoid, but nobody, not even Randall, understood that it had gone from something mild to something acute.

One night I went out to the clubs and got roaring drunk. I ended up on Marietta Street at a massage parlor with a masseuse named Brittany. I had practically crawled in the door, I was so drunk. But they took my credit card and driver's license and didn't turn me away. After the massage, in a moment of paranoia, I thought that Brittany was trying to attack me, so I grabbed her and subdued her. I ran out of that place, jumped in my car and sped home.

The next day, I was so ashamed that I'd assaulted a woman. I knew that they had video cameras in there and wondered if it was all captured on tape. It wouldn't look good. I worried about that day in and day out. The guilt I felt nearly crippled me. Each night that week, I got drunk, trying not to think about it. I was scared that I'd be sent to jail for assault. I wanted to tell somebody, but I couldn't. I went to visit my mom one day to talk to her. She was working from home that day and busy when I got there. I decided to just leave and not interrupt her. As I was going out the door, she called to me and asked why I was leaving so soon. I said it was because she was busy. She said she always had time for me. I was really messed up and wanted to reach out and hug her, but I knew if I did, I'd break down and cry. We both leaned in, but then I turned away. Maybe if I could have brought myself to connect then, things wouldn't have spiraled out of control from there.

That weekend, on January 26th, I went out clubbing again, this time to a spot on Covington Highway, called Primetime. I was hanging out; talking to a girl that I'd met online and had agreed to meet there. I remember telling her to hold on; I needed to get something from my car. When I attempted to come back in, the security guy at the door wanted me to pay a cover charge. I explained to him that I'd just been inside and had gone out to the car to get my wallet. He was rude and obnoxious and insisted that I had to pay. We got into a heated disagreement. The next thing I knew, a cop was slamming me on the ground and arresting me for disorderly conduct when all I had done was ask the security guard to do the right thing.

I spent that night in a jail. I didn't even know where I was. I felt that anything could happen to me and no one would even know. I called my mom, told her the deal, and asked her to rescue me once again. She said not to worry; she thought she knew where I was since I'd been arrested in Dekalb County. She would make some calls and come get me in the morning.

In the morning, she called me back to confirm that she knew where I was and that she was bonding me out.

That jail stay was a nightmare. It lasted less than ten hours, but it seemed like an eternity. I passed the time by calling almost everyone in my cell phonebook who answered. I had normal conversations as though I wasn't sitting in a jail cell. The next day, they didn't give us breakfast. I complained and said it was our right to have three meals. They pulled me out of holding, put me in isolation and fed everybody else except me. By then, I was really hungry because I hadn't had dinner. When I get hungry, I get really agitated and grouchy, so I keep Nutrament on hand to make sure I don't go to that ugly place. There wasn't anything that I could do so I just lay down and used my black corduroy jacket as a pillow. For lunch, they gave us a sandwich that consisted of two slices of bread and a piece of baloney.

Just after noon that Sunday, the bail process was completed and I was free to leave. When I got to the waiting room, I didn't see my mother. So I went outside to look for her, hoping she hadn't left me. She had gone to the car. I was so relieved to see her, but also tired, embarrassed and frustrated. I noticed the jail was on Memorial Drive, in a building that I had passed many times before without even thinking about it.

On the way to the house, I told her about my stay in the jail – about how poorly they treated everyone and the thin baloney and bread sandwich. The sandwich came only after my protests about our rights.

My mother gave me a Nutrament and some bottled water. I gratefully drank it as we drove to 285 and Covington Highway to check on my car. Somewhere in the scuffle with the police officer, I'd lost my key fob. Luckily, there was a spare at my mom's house. I worried about somebody finding the key fob and stealing my car. My mom calmed my fears by saying that nobody would know which car the key fob belonged to, especially since it was lost a block away. I'd left the moon roof open, but the car was safe. We hopped in to head home.

When we got home, she offered me a BLT sandwich made with soy bacon. Hungry as I was, I just couldn't do it, and went into the room to get some rest. I noticed my mail on the dresser and began to sort through it. Among the many attempts to sell me something was a pink card. I opened it to find that it was a Notice of Hearing on Application for Criminal Warrant to determine if there was probable cause for a claim by Brittany. The notice stated that when she tried to get me up and out of the building following the massage session, I grabbed her from behind, put my hand over her mouth and squeezed her in a bear hug. At the time, I was drunk and paranoid out of my mind, but I do remember that I thought that she was trying to hurt me. That's why I jumped up out of my sleep and grabbed her. She had my information from my driver's license, which I'd turned over at the massage parlor. It had taken her two days to file the claim; the appearance date was set for February 7, 2008.

After reading the notice, I became sick to my stomach and felt my life draining from me. I felt a sense of tiredness that I could never have imagined before. One step forward, now two steps back. In my heart, I knew I was going to go to jail. I wondered what the cameras in that massage parlor had picked up. If they captured everything, it would be clear that I had hurt Brittany. My mother kept trying to talk to me through the bedroom door, but I wasn't hearing her. I told her that I was extremely disturbed and was trying to get some rest. I explained the pink card that came in the mail and its contents. I related the events of that evening only a Saturday ago. She said, "Not to worry. We will deal with this, but you know you have to be responsible for your actions." I knew I was responsible for my actions – that was the part that I was worried about. I tried to reach Brittany to talk to her and when I finally got in contact with her to apologize and see if we could settle this outside of court, she said she'd let me know and call me back. I was exhausted after not having slept all night or eaten, but managed to fall asleep for a couple of hours.

When I woke up, I asked my mother if she ever just felt tired. She said yes, but advised me to just keep going. I was supposed to push through and expand – stronger for the experience. I asked her if she wanted to retire early, and she said yes. I was feeling better because I'd made up my mind that I wouldn't have to deal with all this mess. I actually felt refreshed.

My mother talked about how to handle the situation, including retaining a lawyer I'd used before, a Morehouse alumni. It was Super Bowl Sunday and my mom was going to a friend's house to watch the game. She was bringing the sangria and invited me to come along to get my mind off my troubles. I didn't want any part of socializing and quickly rejected the offer.

I asked her to drop me off at my car. As she drove, we had a discussion or, I should say, she talked to me about getting professional help. I said I didn't need to see a shrink. She said I might need some as many people in our family had suffered from alcoholism. Maybe it was something that was triggered in the genes. She said I should stop drinking. I said "Ya think?" Then she started talking about life's struggles and how we are bigger than the life journey we are on and One with Spirit. After this journey, we remember who we are, yet while on earth we forget, so we struggle. I remained quiet, just listening. She had finally realized how much I was struggling. I had hid it well; whenever she asked how I was feeling or if I was happy, I had reassured her that I was fine. Still, in the back of my mind, I thought *isn't a mother supposed to just know?*

Once we got back to my car, I pulled some Tupperware from the trunk that I had been intending to return to my mother. I also had some clothes to donate to a clothing drive she was leading for Samaritan House. I gave those to her, and then I took the jacket off my back and gave that to her, too. She asked me if I was sure that I wanted to give away a perfectly good jacket. I answered yes.

When I got to the house in South West Atlanta, I changed my clothes into my usual casual attire, a green tee-shirt under a maroon Morehouse College hoodie, blue jeans, and my Nike sneakers. I sat and looked back at the events of the past few months. My mother kept calling me, but I didn't answer. Brittany never called me back.

That night, Randall texted me that the Giants had won the Super Bowl and that he wouldn't be home that evening. I texted him back in acknowledgement. Any other time, I could have been excited about a home team win.

I went down to the basement, locked the door, sat on the futon and read the warrants again. I kept reading those two warrants over and over wondering, "How did I get here?" I thought that it was just like with those games back in the community when someone cheated; I didn't want to play anymore. This was not fair. I'd labored in vain, and right now I felt as though everything was moving in slow motion. I was just tired; fatigue had me weary all the time.

If I can't do simple things like pass the CPA or get accepted into the university of my choice, what is the problem with me? I no longer believe I can do anything I want to do. Why can't I seem to focus? This effort of putting on a mask of having it all together every day is wearing me down.

I threw a jump rope up to the beam in the ceiling and pulled. The density of the insulation and the configuration of the ceiling didn't allow it to hold much weight. But I did have the guns, and I went and got the Kimber, returned to the basement and again locked the door behind me.

This is what my life had come to. But I did not have to accept becoming a common criminal. After having spent the last night in jail, I knew I couldn't accept that fate. Just after 10 PM, I pulled out my Blackberry World and texted my mother a message regarding my personal assets: Vanguard - $20k, Citibank - $20k

I put the court documents and my cell phone in the front pocket of my hoodie. Then I leaned a mirror on a rack in front of the futon so that I could be sure to do this correctly. I had found an online video on how not to end up a vegetable. Then I sat down on the futon and updated my note from December 3rd to add my assets, to tell my mom I loved her, and yes, I understood that Life goes on after the death of the body. Also, everyday life goes on. I thought she would understand. But I really wasn't thinking about anyone else; I just wanted to escape the gaping hole of despair that had become my life.

As I sat thinking, I'd have to say that I was a humble guy. Whenever I appeared arrogant, it was just that shadow self that was full of fear and anger. It wasn't the part of me that I wanted to express. When I was balanced, I could make great things happen. I never did anything to give people something to talk about; I did things because I wanted to do them. No one could ever challenge me more than I challenged myself. In fact, I had always been my worst critic and that had driven me to do all the things I'd successfully accomplished. I could accomplish anything, but I'd found out that accomplishments are not everything, especially when the chatter in my brain full of dark thoughts seemed to keep attracting dark circumstances. Maintaining balance was almost impossible. The hurdles seemed higher and more formidable; I'd been crashing through them and the mental pain was excruciating. I couldn't do this anymore.

Looking back, I saw that I'd failed myself. Now I was driven to do the unthinkable. I'd made the ultimate choice. I rested my weary soul without remorse and quit this game of life because it had become more burden than joy. I took the Kimber and fired into the wall about ten feet away as a test shot, then put the gun in my mouth and pulled the trigger.

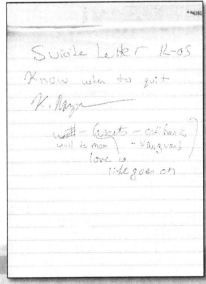

Suicide Letter 12-03

Know when to quit

K. Nazaire
Will to mom (assets – Citibank, - Vanguard)
Love u
Life goes on

Certificate of Death – Khaliyq Nazaire
February 28, 1980 – February 3, 2008

THE END

AFTERWORD

This story is called a tiger's journey because tigers are a breed of integrity. A tiger is a male who is the pride of a family, the one who is believed to be strong because he's never seen crying. He is compassionate, loving, a sincere friend and wise advisor. Strength is his legacy, courage his birthright, as well as his mask. Yet, because of these attributes of manhood, the world can be a heavy burden, for a tiger wants to carry the weight for his loved ones. You may never see his pain because he wants you to see only strength. He also tends to have a great smile. We think our tigers are indefatigable, yet they are not. They see a world that does not reflect their compassion and sometimes end up lost.

We need to teach our young tigers that exterior circumstances may cause pain, but that they are truly only False Evidence Appearing Real—the same fear that causes chaos in this world. To counter this, we can teach and reinforce Divine Law from cradle to grave. Fathers and elders, talk more so that young tigers know they are not alone. It's a rite of passage to face adversity in this world, to transcend limitations and cross that plateau to get to the truth of who we are. We can share knowledge, skills, talent, and information. We care through actions and deeds. Brothers, be friends and your brothers' keepers. Sisters, check a brother's pulse; nurture and, in fact, help to build a brother's strength so that you in turn can lean when you need to.

I say tigers because lions roar and repel. Alpha male pack leaders fight to inherit their space, yet tigers process energy differently through compassion. Young mothers of tiger cubs, sit your sons down regularly; talk with them, feed them their favorite meal and use that time to communicate and share. Fathers, your tigers need to know that you went through the fire and passed through like a phoenix rising to its glory. It's inner strength and tuning in to the Source that gets you through, not a title or career. Hard work alone won't get you there - true success comes with allowing the Source. Your God Self gets you through. Mothers who have been made stronger by tears for their missed tigers now know how to recognize one, and can adopt another son to share with and care for.

A tiger is missed. Let his manner of transition be a guiding message of Love and a call to action. What you choose to do and how you choose to do it is up to you. Just do something in honor of Love.

Khaliyq, your story is shared in honor of your pure love and as a beacon of Light to others.

MEMORY WALL FOR

KHALIYQ NAZAIRE

Cousin Sha-Asia Nazaire
It was supposed to be me and you, cuz. I remember when I used to hate it when you were little and followed me around. Now I wish I could see your face. I know you're with me; I feel you around me, but I will always miss you, always love you.

Godmother Eleanor Ince
Your face, your smile will always stay in my mind and in my heart because you lit up a room when you entered. Your spirit will forever be with us. You will be greatly missed.

Grandma Hurley
Khaliyq was shy and somewhat introverted as a child, but he loved playing tricks on people. Having the upper hand in situations seemed to make him happy even if he was being a little cruel. He hated having to admit that he was wrong or being a loser in a game. At the same time, he took on the role of protector and champion of his friends and family, especially those he considered to be weaker or who were younger than he. He kept his personal feelings to himself and didn't really share his innermost feelings and desires.

K and I had an adversarial relationship. We most often didn't see eye to eye on anything. I'd say red; he'd say blue. At family events, he would not fully participate

A TIGER'S JOURNEY

until someone pulled him into the fray, so to speak. He was very hard on himself. He expected perfection in everything that he did. Unfortunately, he expected the same from everyone else and was often disappointed. I would describe him as determined, proud, neat, hardworking (as long as he didn't have to get his hands dirty), somewhat arrogant. He believed his way was the best way. He thrived on being looked up to and helping people in need.

My happiest time with him was his graduation from Morehouse. I was grinning from ear to ear. He asked me why I was so glad. I explained that his accomplishment could open many doors for him, that it was possible for him to live a better, more prosperous life than I and that I wanted the very best for him in the future. The main thing I learned from him was perseverance – to never give up on your dreams.

His death saddened me deeply. I felt as though a brilliant star had been extinguished. I was disappointed because he might not have realized how much I loved him. I felt that I had failed him in some way. I don't know whether he believed in heaven or hell but I hope he has found the peace that seemed to elude him here on earth. I look forward to being with him once again in the hereafter.

Girlfriend Kiri
    ALL TO MYSELF I find the way
    Back to each golden yesterday,
    Faring in fancy until I stand
    Clasping your ready, friendly hand;
    The picture seems half true, half dream,
    And I keep its color and its gleam

All to myself.
All to myself I hum again
Fragments of some old-time refrain,
Something that comes at fancy's choice,
And I hear the cadence of your voice:
Sometimes 'tis dim, sometimes 'tis clear,
But I keep the music that I hear
All to myself.

All to myself I hold and know
All of the days of long ago
Wonderful days when you and I
Owned all the sunshine in the sky:
The days come back as the old days will,
And I keep their tingle and their thrill
All to myself.

All to myself! My friend, do you
Count all the memories softly, too?
Summer and autumn, winter, Spring,
The hopes we cherished, and everything?
They course my veins as a draft divine,
And I keep them wholly, solely mine
All to myself.

All to myself I think of you,
Think of the things we used to do,
Think of the things we used to say,
Think of each happy, bygone day;
Sometimes I sigh and sometimes I smile,
But I keep each olden, golden while
All to myself

Friend Gordon Johnson

My man, my brother, my friend. Man Khaliyq, why did you have to leave us so early? Who is going to push me to new levels at the job? Who is going to push me to new heights in the gym? Who is going to play ball with me in Harlem on those weekend days in NYC? I love you, brother, and I know one day I will see you again. Until then, I'll keep fighting the fight for both of us. I will never forget you friend/brother. Rest, and make sure when I do see you again, you have that smile ready for me.

Aunt Grace

My wonderful nephew, you are missed more than you could possibly know. I love you for all time.

A NOTE TO SURVIVORS OF
SUICIDE

The tragic end of a life by suicide greatly impacts the lives of the surviving loved ones. There are no words to fully explain the raw emptiness resulting from the loss of a child, sibling, friend or relative to suicide, especially since suicide is preventable if the precipitating disorder is recognized and diagnosed. To begin to share a facsimile of the experience would involve tapping into volatile emotions, emotions that you must allow to come to the surface if you are to heal. The healing practices for those experiencing emotional and mental imbalances are also practices that would benefit suicide survivors.

Those who have witnessed your pain also share your experience. We at the Young Tiger Foundation can be a safe haven as you go through the storm. The rainbow of grace at the end of this storm is the fact that you now have information to share with others and can help prevent another loss.

Young Tiger Foundation
P.O. Box 68
Stockbridge, GA 30281

Web address: *www.youngtigerfoundation.org*
Email: *youngtigerfoundation@gmail.com*

"Why put emphasis on suicide awareness and prevention? Because once a suicide is completed, very sadly, there is no cure. Therefore, we must try to prevent suicide... "
— *Stamp Out Suicide!*

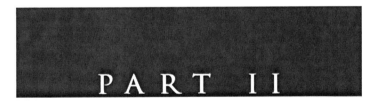

PART II

This material is provided for informational purposes and is not intended to replace the medical advice of a doctor or other health care provider.

CHAPTER 1

BE AWARE

Information leads to empowerment. Suicide is a major, yet preventable health problem. Know the facts. Because most people who commit suicide have a mental disorder (DHHS, 1999b), suicide rates indicate a potential need for mental health care. Statistics from the American Association of Suicidology (the study of suicide) show the rate of suicide among black males between the ages of 15 and 24 increased 83% from the 1980's to the early 1990's. While there has been no further escalation in the rate since the turn of the century, death by suicide is still the third leading cause of death among young black men. Notably, this age group is the only one in which black and white suicide rates run parallel. Also worth noting is the fact that black men are seven times more likely to die by suicide than are black women.

The fact is that the mental dis-ease that can lead to suicide generally stems from chemical imbalances in the brain. With the proper care and maintenance, the person experiencing these imbalances can lead a harmonious life. With this information, you can save a life – that life may be your own or the life of a loved one. The diagnosis of mental dis-ease is highly dependent upon symptoms and behaviors observed and reported by the individual or family. Consequentially, if no one is talking about mental disorder because it is a taboo topic, it is highly unlikely to be diagnosed.

The fact that mental dis-ease is kept in the dark is a primary reason why so many Black American males go untreated. There are many other factors that contribute to the high rate of death by suicide of our youth. The most prominent include:

Mistrust of health professionals – This is based in part on the historically higher-than-average statistics of more severe diagnosis and institutionalization of African Americans with mental illness and previous mistreatment, like the Tuskegee syphilis project. The distrust of health care professionals, combined with the stigma of mental illness, frequently leads African Americans to initially seek mental health support from non-medical sources. Says Henrie M. Threadwell, PhD, of Morehouse School of Medicine, in his article entitled Studies Find Increase in Suicides Among Black Youths: "What's clear is that black communities, health-care professionals and public-health officials must mobilize to meet the challenges presented by this problem."

Cultural barriers between many doctors and their patients -A lack of culturally aware and competent care often results in poor quality care. If a physician is ignorant of the life experiences of a patient, they cannot emphatically deal with the root cause issues. In these cases, an African American physician or healer may better be able to relate to the individual and create a bond of trust. Unfortunately, according to Holzer, Goldsmith and Ciarlo in their 1998 article, "just 2% of the nation's psychiatrists, 2% of the psychologists and 4% percent of social workers, are black."

Reliance on family and religious community - Rather than seeking help from mental health professionals during times of emotional distress, black males generally go to their friends for support. But because of the stigma associated with mental imbalance, they don't pose the issue as a mental health problem. The tendency is to talk about physical problems rather than discuss mental symptoms. Often, a guy will keep the issues to himself and try to mask symptoms with substance abuse or other medical conditions.

Socioeconomic factors – There is also the issue of limited access to medical and mental health care. About 25 percent of African Americans do not have health insurance.

Continued misunderstanding and stigma about mental illness - Many Americans, including black Americans, underestimate the impact of mental disorders. Many believe that symptoms of mental illnesses, such as depression, are "just the blues," a luxury that a strong black male cannot afford. Especially given the mindset in the black community, that to have a mental imbalance makes you weak. We must find ways to get our men to seek help without sacrificing their masculinity. It is not weak to have issues, nor is it weak to seek help with those issues.

Many black American males rely on nonprofessional support or struggle through the dis-ease on their own, but it's clear that the healing needs of our youth are not being met. This is simply because the black community does not address mental health. Yet, because Black Americans often turn to community (family, friends, and clergy) for help, it is important for this group to be aware of risk factors and symptoms and to educate others. As Gina Smallwood, mother of the late Kelvin Smallwood Jones, puts it, "since suicide is the third leading cause of death, the Suicide Hotline Number should be pasted on the phone or refrigerator of every home in the black community, just as you see the poison control number."

Risk factors – Suicidal behavior is complex. Because of this, risk factors vary with age, gender, socioeconomic status, and ethnicity. Other factors include things like: unresolved emotions, exposure to trauma including war and the state of the economy. You may have heard the expression that when America sneezes, Black America catches a cold.

The major risk factors for suicide:

Psychiatric Diagnosis – There are certain psychiatric diagnoses that create a higher risk: depression, bipolar disorder, substance abuse disorders, and personality disorders.

Undiagnosed Depression and other mental disorders – This group is at even greater risk because no medical attention is provided to foster a return to equilibrium and maintenance.

Post-traumatic stress disorders (PTSD) – Survivors of trauma often struggle with nightmares and flashbacks. This could stem from a past event such as childhood sexual abuse or a relatively recent physical occurrence, such as bullying or participating in violent warfare. According to Stephen Soreff, author of the article *Suicide Introduction and Definitions*: "Veterans of Iraq and Afghanistan experience a high rate of PTSD and have a historically high rate of suicide. They have feelings of being damaged and feelings of guilt. As a result, they have a high rate of suicide."

Substance abuse – Excessive use of drugs and/or alcohol, usually initiated to deal with mental dis-ease, can lead to further losses such as a family or job.

Genetics or prior family history of suicide – Studies show a genetic connection to suicidal behavior. If a family member has previously attempted or completed suicide, you are at greater risk of making an attempt yourself.

Prior attempted suicide – If someone previously made a suicide attempt, they are at much greater risk of making a future attempt.

A firearm in the home – Access to firearms is a high risk factor because firearms that are not stored safely provide a lethal means for an attempt.

Sleep deprivation – Deep, refreshing sleep is essential for feeling rested and overall well-being. Lack of sleep can make you feel very sad and could contribute to significant relationship difficulties.

Some antidepressant drugs – Dr. Andrew Mosholder, an expert with America's Food and Drug Administration, reviewed 24 studies involving 4,582 patients taking one of nine different antidepressants. They showed that the drugs nearly doubled the risk of suicide among children and young adults. "The FDA barred him from publishing his findings, but they were leaked to the press in 2004. In 2006, Mosholder's study was published."

Major loss – The loss of a job, death of a loved one (including a pet), major financial loss, or divorce are all significant, stressful events that could preface a suicide attempt.

Contagion by other recent suicides. The "contagion effect", most often seen in adolescents, means that an individual is more likely to attempt suicide if they have recently learned about another suicide, whether it be a relation, friend, or media personality.

Sexual or physical abuse (including bullying) – Studies have shown that children who are repeatedly abused and are abused by members of their immediate family are at greater risk for suicide. Further, those who have been sexually abused are at higher risk than those who were physically abused.

Incarceration – Incarceration is another major risk factor for a suicide attempt. Many people need to be monitored for potential to commit suicide after a recent incarceration.

These risk factors alone do not lead to suicide. These factors, in combination with the changes in brain chemicals called neurotransmitters (with serotonin being the best known), can lead to suicidal behavior. David Esparza, a psychologist and naturopath, explains the role of neurotransmitters in his article, Neurotransmitters, Amino Acids & Mental Health:

> *"A neurotransmitter is a chemical messenger used by neurons to communicate with other neurons. Inside the brain are billions of neurons that are connected by these messengers that transmit electrical impulses from one cell to another, allowing communication and thought to occur in the brain. Certain neurotransmitters, when depleted, may cause you to be easily agitated or angered, experience mild to severe anxiety (or depression) and have sleep problems. Neurotransmitters are 'manufactured' in the brain from the amino acids we extract we extract from foods, and their supply is entirely dependent on the presence of these precursor amino acids."*

Since personality disorder, the name applied to this type of mental dis-ease, is such a huge risk factor, I've provided a descriptive summary from PsychologyNet.org here:

> *Personality disorders are "pervasive chronic psychological disorders, which can greatly affect a person's life. Having a personality disorder can negatively affect one's work, one's family, and one's social life. Personality disorders exist on a continuum so they can be mild to more severe*

in terms of how pervasive and to what extent a person exhibits the features of a particular personality disorder. While most people can live pretty normal lives with mild personality disorders (or more simply, personality traits) during times of increased stress or external pressures (work, family, a new relationship, etc.) the symptoms of the personality disorder will gain strength and begin to seriously interfere with their emotional and psychological functioning.

Those with a personality disorder possess several distinct psychological features including disturbances in self-image; ability to have successful interpersonal relationships; appropriateness of range of emotion, ways of perceiving themselves, others, and the world; and difficulty possessing proper impulse control. These disturbances come together to create a pervasive pattern of behavior and inner experience that is quite different from the norms of the individual's culture and that often tend to be expressed in behaviors that appear more dramatic than society considers usual. Therefore, those with a personality disorder often experience conflicts with other people and vice-versa... treatment focuses on increasing ones coping mechanism and interpersonal skills" as well as addressing diet, sleep and other contributing factors."

Symptoms of Suicide:

Moodiness – Long-lasting sadness and mood swings can be symptoms of depression, a major risk factor for suicide.

General dis-ease – Doubts about self-worth or ability to cope, or simply appearing unhappy and apathetic or showing signs of severe anxiety.

Little or no social contact/pulling away from friends – Choosing to be alone and avoiding friends or social activities are also possible symptoms of depression. This includes the loss of interest or pleasure in activities the person previously enjoyed.

Suddenly having trouble at work or school – Irritability, difficulty concentrating or thinking clearly, distractibility, and indecisiveness can lead to altercations with others, as well as a tendency to lose items.

Recklessness – Potentially dangerous behavior, such as reckless driving, engaging in unsafe sex, and increased use of drugs and/or alcohol might indicate that the person no longer values his or her life.

Anger/Rage – Men tend to externalize their feelings by blaming them on other people, and act out their frustration through anger.

Getting affairs in order – Often, a person considering suicide will begin to put his or her personal business in order. This might include visiting friends and family members, giving away personal possessions, making a will, and cleaning up his or her room or home. Some people will write a note before death by suicide.

Sudden calmness – Suddenly changing behavior, especially calmness after a period of anxiety.

As you can see, there are a myriad of symptoms that could occur in a variety of combinations, confirming how complex suicidal characteristics can be. It is the condition that causes the suicidal thoughts or behavior that should be treated – not just the symptoms. Treating symptoms only provides temporary relief for a disturbance that will resurface. This includes treatment for: bipolar disorder, borderline personality disorder, drug or alcohol dependence and major depression. Combining a mind, body, and spirit treatment approach (e.g., psychotherapy, drugs, herbal remedies, exercise and proper nutrition) with a maintenance program can, over time, facilitate true recovery from mental dis-ease for many individuals and lead to relief for their families.

CHAPTER 2

INDIVIDUALS

Suicidal impulses and depression are signals that you have a health problem. You are outside of your comfort zone because your equilibrium is off-balance. Therefore, natural feelings and emotions meant to serve as guide posts to take actions (anxiety, grief, fear, stress), now become heightened to a degree that is harmful. It is no different from cancer cells multiplying out of control. Therefore, you should not be seeking to end your life, but rather seeking care and help to achieve equilibrium.

Why you? Why do you have a mental imbalance when someone who has been on a similar life path does not? Mental disorders come from many factors. As discussed under Risk Factors, two key factors are neurotransmitter deregulation and environmental factors. Another important factor is genetics. You may have inherited a constitutional vulnerability in that, while one person in the same environment and family may experience mental dis-ease, another may not.

When our vital force energy, or chi, is disturbed and cannot flow freely, we get sick. This disturbance causes energy blockages, which results in imbalance. Without the free flow of energy, Light or happiness is blocked. We can't see the life at the end of the tunnel. This disturbance is not just in the body; it is in the mind, body, and spirit.

You have to treat this trinity. On the bodily level, with the disturbance of the normal functioning of vitality, the brain, like any other organ, gets sick. Depression, paranoia, schizophrenia, bi-polar, and obsessive compulsive disorder all lie on the continuum that is caused by a disturbance in the basic functioning of vitality. Think of your brain as an organ that has a pattern of vibration emanating from a life force. See that pattern as one that is distorted and disconnected. This is what goes on in your brain when you are feeling disempowered.

Mental imbalance or disorder does not only come from life experiences of the mind and the resulting disturbed thought patterns; something as simple as poor digestion of food can also block the free flow of energy.

First, know that are not alone in your experience. Throughout history, some of the greatest thinkers of the world (Sir Isaac Newton, Thomas Edison, and Abraham Lincoln) and creative personalities in the arts (Michelangelo, Thelonious Monk) suffered from mental disorders, and you can be sure that the same is true today.

Some people currently in the public eye include:

Lionel Aldridge - ex Green Bay Packers tight end living with schizophrenia

Joe Budden - hip hop singer who speaks about major depression

Rapper BizzyBone – deals with a schizoaffective disorder

DMX – a rapper who has talked openly about having bipolar disorder

Rickey Williams – a basketball player who lives with social anxiety disorder

Rapper Joe Budden bluntly presents his thoughts of suicide, a permanent solution to a temporary problem like this:

"Why am I meeting so many backstabbers
Why every time that I crash I go faster
Past is a disaster when your house is see through
Learn to close your eyes in case the glass shatters
I'm just saying there's a million more pages
But my stupid ass keeps thinking I'm on the last chapter."

And in another of his songs:

"I got a drug problem that I ain't tending to
Because I got enough problems and my solution is to stuff
Valium
But if something goes wrong with that,
It's back to PCP and so long to rap
I'm depressed lately..."

Mental dis-ease is a common experience in our fragmented society. I want to reiterate that this imbalance is no different from any other dis-ease that can be inherent to anyone's makeup. It's not just the brain that goes awry. It's the mind, body, spirit balance that has lost its equilibrium. A return to balance is what is needed to heal.

For example, with depression, the dis-ease is expressed uniquely in different individuals. While different distortions in brain chemicals lead to varied manifestations of brain chemical imbalance or physiological disturbance, the depression you experience will probably fall into one of three categories noted by Nancy Liebler and Sandra Moss in their book, *Healing Depression the Mind-Body Way*:

> *"Airy depression – caused by low serotonin manifests as a loss of enthusiasm with anxiety as the predominant secondary emotion. The individual has difficulty falling asleep. The driving internal perception is the feeling of being overwhelmed or out of control. The root of the problem is likely to be found in a lack of stability in life patterns. Difficulty sustaining a major life change can be a trigger for this archetype of depression. Nourishing the physiology and stabilizing the nervous system are the main therapeutic techniques.*
>
> *Burning depression – caused by high norepinephrine and/ or dopamine. Here the metabolic processes are blocked. Irritability and frustration are so prevalent that they can often mask a gulf of sadness. The individual's sleep is disrupted because the mind wakes up long before the body is fully rested. The driving internal perception is the feeling of having blocked possibilities. Approaching life with extreme intensity and a pattern of overdoing may be at the root of the problem. To resolve this type of depression, the physiology must be cooled off, literally and figuratively. Decreasing intensity is as essential for recovery as getting deep rest.*
>
> *Earthy Depression – low norepinephrine and/or dopamine. Solidity and stability morph into feelings of being weighed down. Lethargy, lack of interest, and*

being overly sentimental keep the individual feeling stuck. Excessive sleep is a key feature of this archetype of depression. Interventions must address the heaviness experienced at every level in the mind-body. Ayurvedic purification treatments greatly assist in resolving this type of depression."

Healing

You as the experiencer can observe the feelings and thoughts that come about prior to an episode of disease and assist in healing yourself. Healing is never easy. The first step is to forgive yourself and to begin again. This is a lifelong journey and you may find yourself beginning again over and over. That's okay. Forgive yourself for letting yourself down, if you think that is what happened. Most of the time, our actions are really driven by reactions and unexamined forces within us. We don't really have control and are not able to right what is wrong by ourselves because we don't know the root cause of the reaction. We may be reenacting age-old scripts from generations before, yet we don't know how or why. Dig into your family history and you will find stories repeating themselves. You can end that cycle through conscious forgiveness. Forgiveness is the key because it allows you to surrender your ego's need to have life happen just the way you think it should and allow what is currently before you to be; change happens from that space. While there are a myriad of ways to do this, all permanent healing involves allowing one to become balanced and find peace within.

Generally, when you go to a doctor for a mental dis-ease, the first means of healing they will offer is psychotropic drugs. If you choose to use these drugs, be sure that your doctor also informs you of the side effects. Some of them can actually worsen symptoms and enhance your state of imbalance in another area. Your individual healing may require some use of pharmaceutical drugs, yet know that, ultimately, what you require is the return to a state of balance. An understanding of and focus on the root cause of the imbalance is really what is needed. This can be done most effectively through energy work. Note that since mental dis-ease ranges from the mild to acute, these techniques should be used in conjunction with the support and advice of your physician, therapist or licensed counselor.

Dis-ease such as depression is often accompanied by anxiety that causes an individual to have a lot of excess energy, which may manifest as being agitated. In mild cases, simply going for a walk (moving the blocked energy), and focusing one's attention on external factors can begin to move you out of an anxious and dark state of mind, and restore equilibrium. As the blocked energy or chemical imbalance moves up the continuum of severity, more care and effort are needed. Though there are many activities that can contribute to your mental health safety, an effective health maintenance plan is as unique to each individual as your body makeup.

Developing your safety plan:

Medication – Synthetic medications tend to address the symptom rather than the cause and, as mentioned previously, can have many negative side effects. These drugs manage the levels of the three brain chemicals called neurotransmitters: serotonin, dopamine and norepinephrine. Recent research shows the effectiveness of antidepressants to be only slightly more effective than that of a placebo. Yes, the drugs manipulate neurotransmitters, but they do not impact the total being – mind, body and spirit. Since only the symptoms are dealt with, the root cause will eventually manifest itself again in the future.

Homeopathic medicine deals with natural ways of balancing brain chemistry and impacts the mind, body and spirit. Homeopathic drugs are alternative medicines that act as natural remedies; each homeopathic prescription is made specifically to fit the person's unique symptoms. Homeopaths effectively treat depression and other mental dis-ease by helping to get the mental and physical body back into balance. Homeopaths treat the root cause, not the symptom (e.g., depression). Homeopathic healers treat the specific pattern of symptoms that are present in an individual.

Exercise – Use the type of exercise that aligns with your body. It may be martial arts, yoga, breath therapy, muscle building or a combination that will work for you. Try it all, and tailor your own program. Exercise stimulates the physiology and facilitates the free flow of the vital life force, or chi.

Meditation – There are many forms of meditation to still the mind and foster the generation and flow of healing energy. Both moving and stillness meditations are effective, depending on the need. Certainly, if an individual is anxious and cannot sit still, one would not suggest a stillness meditation. In that case, a moving meditation such as martial arts or chi gong would be more appropriate to move stagnant energy.

Yoga – Yoga is known to calm minds and help students deal with stress. ABC –Awareness of your body, Breathing, and Concentration - takes you out of your head, away from internalized thoughts such as hopelessness and despair. Yoga postures work wonders for mild non-clinical depression (defined as depression lasting a day or two), and sufferers who are under the care of a licensed counselor or physician will also benefit.

Breath Therapy – During stressful situations, we tend to hold our breath. This locks in place the tension of the difficult moment. As we repeat this action over time, we are breathing less and less fully and, as a result, do not fully receive oxygen throughout our cells. The result is less energy and decreased vibrancy. Breath Therapy reteaches one how to fully breathe to reduce stress and get more energy.

Chi Gong – This is another form of energy healing that puts emphasis on fluid movement aligned with deep breath work and mindfulness. This allows a person to create new thought patterns by redirecting the mind away from repetitive negative thoughts. By stimulating and clearing the body's energy centers (chakras and meridians), the channels through which energy flows, Chi Gong connects the mind, body and spirit.

Rest – Sleep deprivation, a primary risk factor for suicide, makes both your mind and body less suitable to deal with mental and physical stress. Stress is meant to be a signal to you that something needs to be dealt with. You need to take an action. When the signal is left on, stress turns into negative energy that blocks or imbalances your equilibrium and inhibits sleep. To get proper rest, you may find self-relaxation and hypnosis CD's helpful. Herbal teas, such as chamomile, also support relaxation. It's also helpful to avoid overstimulation before going to bed. This includes stimulating foods and drink as well as media.

Sound therapy – Studies have shown that music stimulates the left brain and the body's natural "feel good" chemicals – dopamine and serotonin. Per Patricia and Rafaele Jourdy in their book *Music to Recharge Your Brain*, the right high frequency sound (or high energy) vibration patterns can enhance brain activity, strengthen neural pathways and balance brain function.

Talk therapy – Talking to a professional can help you to become free of the emotional toxins that cause mental imbalance by escorting you through the unvisited part of yourself that gets pushed into the shadows of your mind. Seeing a psychotherapist does not mean that you are crazy. It does mean that you understand that your mental and emotional health is just as important as your physical heath. Uncovering the areas where you have issues, allows you to develop a plan with the aid of the therapist to return to equilibrium. Again, information is empowering.

In summary, you have to manage your energy to maintain a steady state of equilibrium. Staying well when you have a mental illness is a major factor of an enjoyable life. When you tell your doctor about your overall health, include your mental health in the discussion. Remember you are mind, body and spirit. All aspects of you need to be addressed. That is the only way that you will get the proper care to ensure your mental balance.

To properly manage your energy, you should—

Know your limits – Don't take on so many tasks that you wear yourself out. Scheduling endless tasks, without time to reenergize, drains your energy, leaving you feeling exhausted and depleted. You are no good to yourself or anyone in that condition.

Share your feelings – You'd be surprised at how many people have been where you are. You never know until you start talking about it with someone you trust.

Know your triggers – Once you have a list of the behaviors or symptoms that put you at risk of harm, identify the events, situations, people, thoughts, or feelings that trigger those behaviors or symptoms.

Avoid alcohol and drugs – Often people suffering from mental dis-ease will indulge in alcohol and drugs to numb the pain they are feeling. In Dana Hinder's article on *The Link Between Alcohol and Depression*, she states: "Poor appetite, insomnia, mood swings, feelings of hopelessness, and other common indicators of depression are closely tied to the degree of a person's alcohol consumption."

Watch what you eat – A study conducted at the Psychiatric Clinic, Charles University of Prague showed that patients in their study who had attempted a violent suicide had significantly lower cholesterol levels than patients with non-violent attempts and the control subjects. The authors, J. Vevera, T. Moricinke, and H. Papezova, determined that their findings were "consistent with the theory that low levels of cholesterol are associated with increased tendency for impulsive behavior and aggression and contribute to a more violent pattern of suicidal behavior." They concluded the "data indicate(s) that low serum total cholesterol level is associated with an increased risk of suicide."

Know when to give up an objective – Often, we are forced on by a "quitters never win" mentality. There is a great deal of stigma attached to the word "quit" that connotes failure and weakness. Stubborn persistence may be an asset in some situations, yet when success in an area has become your indicator of personal self-worth and you are subsequently feeling unworthy, quitting or stopping to reassess your priorities and redirect your actions can be the best thing that you can do.

Reconnect to a sense of purpose – Therapy alone won't make you want to live. You have to find a reason for living. Often, if one does not have a goal - something to work for and look forward to - they will just drift through life unfulfilled. Additionally, we see the "walking wounded" sleep walking through their own lives every day. These are people who lost their vibrant energy to some tragic or traumatic event and, as a result, have very little connection to present life. Having a reason to live comes from a connection with life purpose, a connection to the present moment and your soul. It doesn't mean that everything in life is alright. It simply means that you can move through life's issues because you are focused on a higher purpose.

If you get to the point of crisis:

Crisis is defined as a "mental health emergency" (e.g., your urges to harm get to the point that you are at immediate risk of committing suicide or for harming someone else). Go to a hospital if there is one nearby, or call an emergency phone number on hand. In the U.S., call the National Suicide Hotline: 1-800-273-8255.

Before you can ever get to this point, we ask that you agree to and sign the No Suicide Agreement below:

No Suicide Agreement

I _____ make a pact with my Self and all humanity that I will not purposefully do harm to myself or another. I will not let the feelings of despair and hopelessness overtake me. Taking my life is not a solution to the pain I am feeling. I will accept the despair as a feeling based on a current situation and not make it a statement about me or my entire future. On my life journey I will have experiences leading to states of frustration, anger and hopelessness. If I get to the point of despair, I will try to step out of the unforgiving past, stop thinking about a bleak future and deal with only getting through the present moment without judgment of my challenges. When I cannot find equilibrium myself, I will get help before taking another step. Once I have restored my balance, I can look at the situation through clearer eyes and make a sound decision.

Signed: _____
Date: _____

Your life is the only one that matters at this point. You are the center of your universe. You owe it to yourself to move through the next moment, the next hour, and the next day with focus on your well-being. Get help, until you are able to stop the self-sabotage and to find balance on your own. Many have dedicated their lives to helping you, including the Young Tiger Foundation. To find out more about the Young Tiger Foundation go to *www.youngtigerfoundation.org*.

CHAPTER 3

FAMILY AND FRIENDS

You can help. Ladies, help your husband, boyfriend, father, brother or son by paying attention to his emotional state. Ask him how he feels, not how he is doing. He could be doing fine outwardly and be on the brink of despair inwardly. He may be at risk for suicidal behavior and not get treatment for many reasons, as stated previously in the section of risk factors. The primary reasons:

- He believes nothing will help.
- He does not want to tell anyone he has problems.
- He thinks it's a sign of weakness to ask for help.
- He does not know where to go for effective help.

Many times, we see signs of imbalance and write these symptoms off as a personality trait, rather than a personality disorder. Often things do work out; we all go through cycles of imbalance. Yet, when small signs continue to occur, it's up to you to offer support and encourage your loved one to seek professional help. Let them know that with the right combination of treatment, they can lead normal lives just as a cancer or AIDS patient can.

You must also realize that depression and other disorders are very real imbalances. Your loved one cannot "just snap out of it." In the case of the loss of a family member or job, the disturbed individual cannot "just get over it." You must understand that the mental imbalances that lead to suicide are very real illnesses that require treatment.

What does not help:

- Trying to tell the person how well off they are compared to others,
- Minimizing their feelings,
- Arguing with them,
- Judging the situation,
- Trying to deal with a suicidal person without professional help.

What should you do if someone you know is talking about taking their own life?

First and foremost, take the threat seriously! Then:

- Do not leave the person alone. If possible, ask for help from friends or other family members.
- Ask the person to give you any weapons he or she might have. Take away sharp objects or anything else that the person could use to hurt his or herself.
- Try to keep the person as calm as possible.
- Call 911 or take the person to an emergency room and, ultimately,
- Become trained as a gatekeeper, so you will understand the signs of distress and deal with them accordingly.

Paul Quinett, PhD, describes the role of gatekeeper training in his Question Persuade and Refer (QPR) Theory Paper as, "The goal of gatekeeper training is straightforward: to enhance the probability that a potentially suicidal person is identified and referred for assessment and care *before* an adverse event occurs. As population-based approach, the greater the percentage of the members of a given community who are trained to successfully recognize and refer its suicidal members, the fewer suicide-related adverse events should occur … *The person most likely to prevent you from taking your own life, is someone you already know.*"

Always take suicide attempts and threats seriously. Statistics show that about one-third of people who attempt death by suicide will try again within a year. In addition, about ten percent of people who threaten or attempt death by suicide will eventually kill themselves. This person needs mental health care right away. Do not dismiss them as someone just trying to get attention.

As one individual heals, the whole of humanity begins to shift. Sooner or later, we've made an impact. Suicide rates will decrease and eventually, like polio, can become virtually nonexistent. There will always be cycles of disease; through learning suicide prevention and awareness techniques and with the knowledge that mental, physical and spiritual balance is the key, you can detect imbalance in another or know when to get help for yourself. We are a village; we need each other to maintain equilibrium for ourselves and the planet.

PART III

APPLYING THE INFORMATION

L et's get families, schools and book clubs talking about spreading the word about a preventable cause of death. Now that you have read *Leaping Through the Hurdles of Life*, as well as the summary of personality disorder and depression, here is a practical opportunity to apply what you learned by correlating the risk factors and symptoms to Khaliyq's life. Hindsight is twenty-twenty, and you can clearly identify applicable risk characteristics and traits in Khaliyq. While no one person could see the fully shattered picture, fragments of clear warning signs were definitely available to many. Answering these questions will help you be able to identify these factors in someone else's life.

Where did the first signs of Khaliyq's personality disorder appear?

In what ways does this imbalance show up?

Why do you think no one knew how bad the situation was?

How specifically was the sense of helplessness masked?

How could the pieces of information have been shared/ pulled together?

How were Khaliyq's personality disorders written off as personality traits?

Life is a journey, where we tumble and fall freely. We can survive anything, if we have the information that allows us to make better choices, along with a village of support. Since it is impossible to know the burden that anyone is carrying, we should be kind to all. You never know when that smile, or letting someone ahead of you in the line or on the road, will make a difference to someone who just needs a sign of Grace.

MANY THANKS

The life story of Khaliyq Nazaire was narrated based on firsthand knowledge of the author, friends, family and relatives, as well as the meticulous documentation maintained by Khaliyq. Special thanks to Kaliel Ali, Randall Frazier, Audrey Hurley, Jamari Haynes, Gordon Johnson II, Charles Jones, Keith Jones and Xavier Lancaster for sharing their stories and their love.

Thanks to the final editors, Lemuel LaRoche and Britney Robertson for truly feeling the story and understanding the message being shared. Your direction and encouragement helped make this memoir a clear statement to all.

Thanks to Rev. Rowena Silvera, the Sunday Soul Diva, for channeling the "Khaliyqism" never bow to false gods.

Thanks to my niece, Sha-Asia, for being my shadow in those early days.

Thanks to my personal coach, Rev. Dr. Dee Adio-Moses, for pushing me to deliver this message that so many people are waiting to hear.

Related Resources, Information and Professional Organizations to look into:

QPR Theory http://www.qprinstitute.com/theory.html

Sound Therapy: Music to Recharge your Brain by Patricia and Rafaele Joudry

Website: www.soundtherapyinternational.com

Mind Management Training, Dr. Mark Armstrong, Ahimki Center for Wholeness, www.ahimki.net

Healing Depression the Mind-Body Way, creating happiness with meditation, yoga, and Ayurveda, by Nancy Liebler, Ph.D, and Sandra Moss, M.S.P.H

CPSIA information can be obtained at www.ICGtesting.com
Printed in the USA
LVOW120723040912

297257LV00002B/1/P

9 780984 833504